Sweden's Pandemic Story: Covid-19, A Chronology 2020–23

Graeme D. Eddie

Sweden's Pandemic Story: Covid-19, A Chronology 2020–23

Foolhardy, Exceptional, or Just Principled?

PETER LANG
New York · Berlin · Bruxelles · Chennai · Lausanne · Oxford

Bibliographic information published by the Deutsche Nationalbibliothek. The German National Library lists this publication in the German National Bibliography; detailed bibliographic data is available on the Internet at http://dnb.d-nb.de.

Library of Congress Cataloging-in-Publication Data
Library of Congress Control Number: 2025042804

Cover image: PalSand. Sourced from Shutterstock, image no. 1680603880.
Cover design by Peter Lang Group AG

ISBN 978-3-0343-6077-7 (Print)
ISBN 978-3-0343-6078-4 (E-PDF)
ISBN 978-3-0343-6079-1 (E-Pub)
DOI 10.3726/b23075

Published by Peter Lang Publishing Inc., New York (USA)

info@peterlang.com - www.peterlang.com

This publication has been peer reviewed.

Contents

Acknowledgements

Writing for most of this work, *Sweden's Pandemic Story: COVID-19, A Chronology 2020–23. Foolhardy, Exceptional, or Just Principled?* was carried out in Dunbar, Scotland, during the worst COVID-19 pandemic years.

For this book and an earlier title, *Swedish Foreign Policy, 1809–2019: A Comprehensive Modern History* (Peter Lang, New York, 2020), and for several articles for *The World Today*, a journal of the Royal Institute for International Affairs (RIIA, London), research effort had been enhanced through acquisition of Swedish language skills over many decades, particularly reading skills.

This had enabled access to original Swedish-language government, parliamentary, ministerial, departmental, and journalistic sources. In this regard, recognition is given to the language instruction given at the Helsingborg locale of the Folk University of Sweden in the 1970s, and by lecturing staff during the 1980s at the Scandinavian Studies Departments at Aberdeen and Edinburgh Universities, and to the teaching staff at Linköping University. Research and study in Sweden in these earlier decades was assisted by the Swedish Institute.

Importantly too, special thanks are given to Brian Walsh for his continued encouragement and patience during the research and writing process leading to this work on the Swedish pandemic experience.

The cover illustration, showing a mask-wearing Astrid Lindgren (1907–2002) was sourced from Shutterstock (Image no. 1680603880) and is the work of PalSand. Lindgren, the renowned Swedish author whose pen created *Pippi Långstrump*, or *Pippi Longstocking*, and *Alla vi barn i Bullerbyn*, had been featured on a Swedish Kronor 20 note issued in 2015 (without the mask of course).

Graeme D Eddie
September 2025
Dunbar
East Lothian
Scotland

Acronyms and Abbreviations

ACT-A	Access to COVID-19 Tools Accelerator
BBC	British Broadcasting Corporation
CCDC	Chinese Centre for Disease Control and Prevention
CSG	Coronaviridae Study Group
CVST	Cerebral venous sinus thrombosis
DN	Dagens Nyheter
EBU	European Broadcasting Union
ECB	European Central Bank
EEA	European Economic Area
EEAS	European External Action Service
EMA	European Medicines Agency
EU	European Union
EUR	Euro/s
FAO	Food and Agricultural Organization
FHI	Folkehelseinstituttet (Norway)
GAVI	Global Alliance for Vaccines and Immunizations
GDP	Gross domestic product
HIV	Human immunodeficiency virus
ICTV	International Committee on Taxonomy of Viruses
ICU	Intensive care unit
IPCR	Integrated Political Crisis Response
IVO	Inspektionen för vård och omsorg, or Health and Social Care Inspectorate
KU	Konstitutionsutskottet, or parliamentary Standing Committee on the Constitution
KVA	Kungliga Vetenskapsakademien, or Royal Swedish Academy of Sciences

LR	Lärarnas Riksförbund, or the National Union of Teachers
MERS	Middle East respiratory syndrome
mRNA	Messenger ribonucleic acid
MSB	Myndigheten för samhällsskydd och beredskap, or Civil Contingencies Agency
MUF	Moderata ungdomsförbundet, or Moderate Youth League
NATO	North Atlantic Treaty Organization
NIH	National Institutes of Health
NIPH	Norwegian Institute of Public Health, or Folkehelseinstituttet, FHI
OECD	Organisation for Economic Co-operation and Development
ONS	Office for National Statistics (UK)
PCC	Post-COVID-19 condition, or 'long-COVID'
PHEIC	Public Health Emergency of International Concern
PPE	Personal protective equipment
PRAC	Pharmacovigilance Risk Assessment Committee
SAGE	Scientific Advisory Group for Emergencies
SALAR	Swedish Association of Local Authorities and Regions, or Sveriges Kommuner och Regioner, SKR
SARS	severe acute respiratory syndrome
SCB	Statistics Sweden (Statistikmyndigheten, SCB), formerly Statistika centralbyrån or Central Bureau of Statistics
SEK	Swedish kronor
SIDA/Sida	Swedish International Development Corporation Agency
SIPRI	Stockholm International Peace Research Institute
SKR	Sveriges Kommuner och Regioner
SOU	Statens Offentliga Utredningar, or Swedish Government Official Reports
SSI	Denmark's State Serum Institute, or Statens Serum Institut
SVA	Statens Veterinärmedicinska Anstalt, or National Veterinary Institute
SvD	Svenska Dagbladet
SVT	Sveriges Television, Swedish Television
TAG-VE	Technical Advisory Group on SARS-CoV-2 Virus Evolution
UN	United Nations
UNEP	UN Environment Programme
VAT	Value added tax
WHA	World Health Assembly
WHO	World Health Organization
WOAH	World Organization for Animal Health
WTO	World Trade Organization

Swedish Regions & Principal Towns & Cities (2020)

In 2020, the first year of COVID-19, the population of Sweden was 10,327,589. European Union countries close to Sweden in size were Belgium 11.5 million, Greece 10.7 million, Czechia 10.6 million, Portugal 10.4 million, and Hungary 9.7 million.

In the following table, listed from the Arctic north to the Baltic south, are Sweden's 21 devolved regions (*regioner*) after the most recent adjustment of the country's administrative divisions and nomenclature in January 2020, with some of the larger communities (towns and cities) in each. The regions organize, fund, and deliver health care, with the government setting policy, and the National Board of Health and Welfare (*Socialstyrelsen*) developing standards:

Region Norbotten	Luleå, Piteå, Kiruna, Boden
Region Västerbotten	Umeå, Skellefteå, Lycksele
Region Jämtland Härjedalen	Östersund, Strömsund, Åre
Region Västernorrland	Sundsvall, Örnsköldsvik, Härnösand
Region Gävleborg	Gävle, Sandviken, Hudiksvall
Region Dalarna	Borlänge, Falun, Avesta
Region Värmland	Karlstad, Arvika, Kristinehamn
Region Uppsala	Uppsala, Enköping, Knivsta
Region Västmanland	Västerås, Arboga, Fagersta
Region Örebro	Örebro, Karlskoga, Kumla
Region Stockholm	Stockholm, Huddinge, Nacka
Region Södermanland	Nyköping, Eskilstuna, Katrineholm
Region Västra Götaland	Gothenburg (Göteborg), Borås

Region Östergötland	Linköping, Norrköping, Motala
Region Jönköping County	Jönköping, Nässjö, Tranås
Region Kalmar County	Kalmar,Västervik, Oskarshamn
Gotland Municipality	Visby
Region Halland	Halmstad, Varberg, Kungsbacka
Region Kronoberg	Växjö, Ljungby, Älmhult
Region Blekinge	Karlskrona, Karlshamn
Region Skåne	Malmö, Helsingborg, Lund, Kristianstad

In 2020, the most populace Swedish region was Region Stockholm including the capital Stockholm with 2,391,990 people, followed by Region Västra Götaland including the second city of Gothenburg, with 1,734,443, then Region Skåne including the third largest city Malmö with 1,389,336, followed by Region Östergötland with 467,158, and then Region Uppsala with 388,394 people. The top three most populace regions accounted for 5.51 million, nearly half the population of Sweden, and the top five accounted for 6.37 million.[1,2]

1 'Population on 1 January', Data Browser, Eurostat, <https://ec.europa.eu/eurostat/databrowser/view/tps00001/default/table?lang=en&category=t_demo.t_demo_pop>

2 'Population density per sq km by region, sex, observations and year', 2020, Statistical Database, *Statistics Sweden* (*Statistikmyndigheten*, *SCB*), <https://www.statistikdatabasen.scb.se> accessed 16 May 2025.

Introduction

Sweden the 'Outrider', Sweden the Maverick

With a chair appointed in 2021, and terms of reference received in 2022, the independent and public UK COVID-19 Inquiry was set up to examine the UK response to and impact of the novel coronavirus pandemic that had arrived in Europe in early-2020, and to learn lessons for the future. Public hearings began in June 2023 and would continue into 2026.[1]

The pandemic had affected everyone, and it still has a lasting impact on many. The inquiry invited the public to share how the pandemic had impacted their lives, whether they had run a business, been self-employed, been furloughed, had needed financial support. Every story had mattered.[2]

Some years on from 2020, the individual experience – the stories that mattered – the national experience, the continent-wide experience, and the global experience remained of interest. Indeed, the UK COVID-19 Inquiry had been concerned to understand the response taken to the pandemic in Sweden – considered by many to have been an unorthodox one – and Anders Tegnell, the country's former state epidemiologist had been called to present a witness statement in October 2023.[3] Sweden had experienced its own pandemic inquiry *Coronakommissionen* appointed in June 2020, and a final report was presented in February 2022.

Sweden's national pandemic story was a tale worthy of the telling. As the title suggests, *Sweden's Pandemic Story: COVID-19, A Chronology 2020–23. Foolhardy, Exceptional, or Just Principled?* relates how the country and its people were affected by the pandemic from its arrival in late-January 2020, and over the worst of the crisis, a period reported on by *Coronakommissionen* in February 2022. The pandemic would not end then, of course, and even today people could still catch COVID-19 even if fully or partially vaccinated – breakthrough infection – or had caught the virus before. Indeed, into 2025, the 'Nimbus' (NB 1.8.1) co-circulating variant, a descendent lineage of the Omicron-variant, had shown itself to be growing as a proportion of all coronavirus cases internationally, and was being monitored by the World Health Organization (WHO). But for all that, it is acknowledged that much which has been described in the book here, and much that had been experienced 2020–23, has already passed into national folk memories, no longer part of the everyday or day-to-day.

On 11 March 2020, when the rapidly spreading novel coronavirus, COVID-19, was declared a global pandemic by the WHO it had already begun to affect the lives of everyone in the world. Mitigation measures closed schools, colleges, and universities, and shut down assembly lines and processes. The measures closed the workplaces of nearly everyone except for key workers in food and medicine production, and for those involved in food retail, health and social care provision, and transport. They caused shortages in supply and panic buying, postponed sports, cultural, political, and religious events, and brought about worldwide social and economic disruption and recession.

Week by week, the consequences of the pandemic and of containment and mitigating measures put in place by governments would affect people in different ways. It would colour and mark a generation, and its future chances. World economic output was at least 7 per cent lower than it would otherwise have been, amounting to the biggest slump since the Second World War.[4]

For Sweden, COVID-19 became the nation's, the people's, and the government's most difficult crisis since the Second World War. Nothing comparable to the pandemic had been experienced since 1945 and no external event had such a huge effect on the lives of so many individuals, nor for so long.[5]

Three years on from the first arrival of COVID-19 in Sweden, a regional population-based study – the Linköping COVID-19 study – which included all patients hospitalised due to COVID-19 during the first pandemic wave, reported that four months after discharge from hospital, 40 per cent of patients were experiencing 'long-COVID', or post-COVID-19 condition, PCC. These were 'persisting symptoms and activity/participation limitations' which even twenty-four-months after discharge included cognitive, sensorimotor, and debilitating fatigue symptoms.[6]

Indeed, a wider Nordic study of persons with COVID-19 from Iceland, Sweden, Denmark, and Norway, indicated that physical symptoms of shortness of breath, chest pain, dizziness, headaches, and low energy/fatigue persisted up to twenty-seven-months after diagnosis.[7] A small number of Swedes had still been on sick leave one year after their COVID-19 diagnosis, indicating a 'need for long-term follow-ups to identify people who might benefit from targeted vocational rehabilitation'.[8]

PCC had implications for the individuals themselves, their national health and social services, productivity, and the labour force. However, even now, 'long-COVID' remained poorly understood 'with a lack of consensus around its specific definition'.[9]

As is well known, Sweden's approach to tackling COVID-19 had been a unique one, often described as an 'experiment', and various elements of that approach and how it affected the ordinary Swede are considered in this work.[10] It had been a strategy 'met with both harsh criticism and some admiration, at home and abroad', wrote Social Democrat Prime Minister Stefan Löfven in his autobiography.[11] The approach had been described by scientists, politicians, and journalists alike, as risky, brave, and sometimes 'foolhardy'. Sweden was expressing its 'exceptionalism'. Sweden was an 'outrider', an 'outlier'. Sweden had achieved pariah status.

The criticism and admiration – a fascination in a way – had been particularly focussed on the decision to keep nurseries and primary schools open, lack of national lockdown, and no mask-wearing. Hard lockdowns, keeping children at home, the wearing of masks, and a range of regulations and restrictions in some countries were, of course, what typified the experience of most countries in Europe and around the world, and which had not been endured since the Second World War.

Not so in Sweden though, and because of that the country was put under the spotlight in a manner and an experience not uncommon over the last eighty years. Western critics had in the past pointed to Sweden and its alcoholism, suicides, divorce rates, rapes, morality, Islamization, no-go areas, crime, and immigration. Those in praise of Sweden, and those mocking of the country, would point to 'Swedish exceptionalism', a sort of nationalist ideology,[12] in areas such as welfare politics, public administration, international relations, and development aid[13] – in these, it profiled itself as superior and the moral superpower, went the narrative.[14] Critics had pitted Anders Tegnell, chief epidemiologist at the public health agency, and 'Swedish exceptionality' against domestic and foreign experts to generate conflicting narratives in the news. And part of the conflict 'involved people's trust in politicians'.[15]

But had there ever really been a unique Swedish way of dealing with COVID-19? Hadn't Sweden shared the same goals as every other country? Hadn't Sweden worked with the same challenges as other countries? Hadn't Sweden simply used the same tools as every other country, but had utilized them in a different way and in a way that suited it best?

Some five years on from draconian lockdowns elsewhere, much reflection had taken place over the lockdown legacy, reflection that will doubtless be repeated as succeeding significant anniversaries are reached and national stories revisited. With public and scholarly interest in the intriguing and poorly understood Swedish approach to the pandemic, and Sweden's experience of it, this work is an attempt to rummage through the, at times, bare falsehood, myth, misrepresentation, misunderstanding, and misconception around that approach.

It observes that:

- excluding formal lockdowns, information from the public health agency and local authorities had differed little from what citizens elsewhere in the EU had been given
- it had not been Sweden engaging in a reckless, unprecedented pandemic experiment, but much of the world, and without any evidence of the sense of implementing drastic lockdowns
- while in the first few weeks of the pandemic Sweden indeed had recorded more deaths per million in a rolling seven-day average than in other Nordic countries, on a number of days the UK had overtaken it
- on the measure of daily new cases per million on a rolling seven-day average in Europe, six months after the WHO announcement of the public health emergency, Sweden had recorded 21.93, while Belgium, for example, had recorded 45.13
- the creation of a negative image of Sweden over its COVID-19 strategy had served as a useful tool abroad, deflecting public attention from local shortcomings
- although herd immunity had never been in sight in Sweden, statistically, and had been regarded only as a possible side effect of strategy, it was nevertheless a respectable concept in epidemiology with, after all, herd immunity being the aim of mass vaccination
- by September 2020 the Swedish R-number had dropped below 1, while across all four nations of the UK around the same time, the R-number ranged between 1.3 and 1.6
- by autumn of the first year of the pandemic, measures introduced had made Sweden seem more like the rest of Europe
- on the measure of daily new confirmed deaths per million (on a rolling seven-day average) at end-October 2020, Belgium had recorded 10.91, while Sweden had recorded 0.07
- into the first weeks of winter 2020, the UK of Boris Johnson could be described as 'outlier', and indeed into 2021, the UK had one of the highest rates of infection in Europe
- by autumn 2021, Sweden had recorded one of the lowest rates in Europe of daily new confirmed cases per million in a rolling seven-day average
- into October 2021, the spread of COVID-19 infection in Sweden had been significantly lower than in almost all other European countries and certainly those in Sweden's near neighbourhood of Baltic and Nordic Europe

- by the end of 2021, while Sweden still compared badly with its Nordic neighbours, comparisons with similar sized countries in Europe, on the measure of cumulative deaths per million, showed that Sweden was far from the 'outlier' with 1,506.87 deaths per million compared to 3,368.81 deaths per million in Czechia which was only slightly larger in population
- on the matter of 'counting,' authorities administering population registration (deaths) automatically checked the lists of people who were infected, so everyone who died and had tested positive for the virus was counted as a COVID-19 death, even if they died from a heart attack or a fall, meaning that Sweden reported many who died 'with' COVID-19, not 'of' COVID-19

The book observes too that there had been room for positive acknowledgement of the Swedish approach, with the country emerging from the first year of pandemic with a smaller increase in its overall mortality rate than most European countries. Also, by March 2025, cumulative deaths from coronavirus in Sweden amounted to 28,670, while in Czechia the figure was 43,807. Overall, surely the Swedish stance had shown its merits.

Finally, it observes that neither a run of political crises throughout 2021, nor the state of health and social care during the pandemic, nor even the war in Ukraine, had figured in the minds of Swedish voters during the 2022 General Election campaign.

While the focus of the work is clearly Sweden and the pandemic – offering what it says on the tin – in many respects it is the story of COVID-19 in the UK, the USA, and the Nordic region as well, statistical comparisons with neighbours Iceland, Finland, Denmark, and Norway frequently shown. It describes the crisis involving Danish mink and anxieties over the mutated virus having been transmitted to humans, and the subsequent culling of this farmed animal in Denmark. It looks at Iceland which, after virtually ridding itself of the virus, suffered from an unexpectedly ferocious wave over summer 2020. The story also takes us beyond the Nordic region to India and the onslaught of the virus there.

In the main though, it is a narrative about Sweden and its own crisis, taking us to the arrival of the novel coronavirus and the mitigation measures put in place, and to the scientific counterattack which began in laboratories across the world right from the very start. In these first few weeks and months, most of normal life remained open and the wearing of masks was not required. People were assumed to take their own individual precautionary measures without a mandate from authorities.[16] 'To keep society largely open', wrote Löfven, the government had to 'rely on the judgement' of Swedes. Throughout the pandemic, the policy 'was to appeal to their common sense and ability to be responsible citizens'.[17]

Swedish mortality is considered in the work, as well as the social and cultural differences (structural factors) affecting the death rate. It was seen in the initial phase of the pandemic in spring 2020 that coronavirus affected the Swedish population unequally, with excess mortality among the socio-economically vulnerable, many of whom had a migrant background.[18] Excess mortality among the migrant population notwithstanding, a study conducted in the first year of the pandemic March 2020 to February 2021 found that in Sweden 'high excess mortality was spread across' the country with 'little or no regional clustering of excess mortality'.[19] Did this indicate similar standards of care within health and social care across the country, rural and urban?

Among the reasons for excess mortality among the socio-economically vulnerable were the different conditions in which people in Sweden lived. The means of limiting social contact and distance differed, depending on the number of people in the household and in the local area, the possibility of working from home, and the ability to avoid public transport. Individuals who, due to these structural factors, were at high risk of infection, also performed a significant part of the care of the most vulnerable in society (looking after older members of their own family in the same household, or in employment in the care sector).[20]

The R-rate in Sweden is given focus too, along with other statistical data including case numbers. It visits the question of mask wearing, vaccines and vaccination, virus variants, spikes in the number of cases, the re-opening of the country, and the donation of millions of vaccine doses to low-and middle-income countries through the COVAX global vaccine initiative.

The book considers domestic criticism of the risky Swedish strategy as well as its defence. It seemed to many that decisions had been left to 'a narrow, self-perpetuating cadre of public health authorities' in an approach – an anomaly – that stood out, neither shutting down nor imposing 'more than mild restrictions'. Sweden's 'public health authorities had preened themselves in the unexpected glow of attention', ignoring science as it developed. As for the coalition government, it had been 'feeble' and 'provided only lacklustre leadership'.[21] And the opposition? Heavily critical of the scale of mortality among the elderly, Jimmie Åkesson, the Sweden Democrat leader, had used words like 'massacre' to describe the Swedish death rate, and said that it had been a 'slaughter of its own population'. Ebba Busch, the Christian Democrat leader, had 'accused the government of deliberately allowing the spread of the infection'. The criticism of both was described by Löfven as 'vulgar rhetoric' and that these 'were among the exceptions in the corona debate'.[22] Just how great had the political opposition been from the opposition parties in parliament, the *Riksdag*? And in the municipalities where the opposition Moderates were largely in control, how had they performed?

A chapter of the work is given over to consideration of the foreign attacks against the Swedish approach. It seemed that when choices had been made about pandemic strategies in the earliest weeks of the crisis – a time when end results could not have been known – many politicians and journalists around the world, not least in the United States, had attacked Sweden fiercely for choosing an unusual and more liberal path, avoiding draconian lockdown. And their own paths? For whatever reason, and for whatever inspiration that took them to their decisions, almost every country in the world, at the same time, chose to implement long, hard lockdowns. Looking at Sweden, they saw the contrast that they would rather not have seen, undermining their own lockdown mantra of having had 'no choice' in adopting it and forcing them to explain to their own people, why they had done it. In 'lambasting Sweden' they 'hid their own insecurities'.[23] Just what was it about Sweden? Why was 'Sweden-bashing' the often-used tool of politicians on the American right? Why were American leaders happy to sacrifice the goodwill of Sweden? Had it something to do with Sweden being a country of progressive politics and openness, and a positive role model for many?

Considered too in the book is the *Coronakommission* which had been set up with the formal remit of evaluating the measures taken by the government, administrative authorities, and municipalities to limit the spread of the virus and to examine the effects of its spread. The commission had presented its final report in 2022. What were its findings? Who was held accountable? Where had the blame been laid? Did it matter anyway, for by the time the final report of *Coronakommissionen* had been published in 2022 the major actors in the drama had either retired, resigned, or moved on. What had the opposition proposed as the best strategy against COVID-19? What had it suggested as the best way forward?

Finally, while international comparisons of the COVID-19 experience were difficult, and the long-term effects of the lockdowns put in place across the world still unknown, the book nods towards how, on many measures – economic, school closures and learning loss, vaccination, studies on suicide, domestic abuse – there were indications that Sweden had done much better than other countries during the pandemic.[24]

Sweden…foolhardy or exceptional, pariah or paragon?[25] Let the story begin.

Chapter 1 will focus on the origin of coronavirus and its arrival in Sweden, as well as the approach taken by the government and public agencies, the measures put in place to slow it down, and the scientific fightback. Why had schools been kept open? As the crisis developed, what information and advice did the public health agency and local health authorities give to Swedes? Was it in any way different to what was given to the citizens of other EU countries? What had been the intent of the Swedish strategy? What did the mitigations measures cost, initially? Would the EU invest in a post-COVID plan?

Notes

1 Website for background and terms of reference of the UK COVID-19 Inquiry, and detail concerning 'Every story matters', <https://covid19.public-inquiry.uk/documents/terms-of-reference/> and <https://covid19.public-inquiry.uk/every-story-matters/>accessed 15 January 2025.

2 Ibid., 'Every story matters'.

3 Witness statement of Professor Anders Tegnell. Statement No.1, Exhibit AT/001, UK Covid-19 Inquiry, 2 October 2023, https://covid19.public-inquiry.uk/wpcontent/uploads/2023/12/18145343/INQ000283502.pdf accessed 16 January 2025.

4 'The plague year', The Economist, Vol. 437, No. 9225, 19 December 2020, p. 17.

5 Löfven, Stefan. i samarbete med Ulrika Knutson. *Svetsare och statsminister*, 2024, p. 170.

6 Wahlgren, Carl *et al.* 'Two-year follow-up of patients with post-Covid-19 Condition in Sweden: a prospective cohort study', *The Lancet Regional Health – Europe*, Volume 28, 100595, May 2023, <https:doi.org/10.1016/jlanepe.2023.100595> accessed 21 January 2025.

7 Shin, Qing *et al.* 'Covid-19 illness severity and 2-year prevalence of physical symptoms: an observational study in Iceland, Sweden, Norway and Denmark', *The Lancet Regional Health – Europe*, Volume 35, 100756, October 2023, <https://doi.org/10.1016/j.lanepe.2023.100756> access 21 January 2025.

8 Abzhandadze, Tamar *et al.* 'Sick leave one year after Covid-19 infection: a nationwide cohort study during the first wave in Sweden', *Scientific reports*, 14, 572 (2024), 5 January 2024, <https://doi.org/10.1038/s41598-50413-9> accessed 21 January 2025.

9 Gonzalez, Ana Espinosa. and Elina Suzuki, 'The impacts of long Covid across OECD countries' OECD Health Working Papers No. 167, 13 June 2024, <https://dx.doi.org/10.1787/8bd08383-en> accessed 21 January 2025.

10 The reader can do no worse than turn to these studies of Sweden's pandemic strategy: Anderberg, Johan, *The Herd: How Sweden chose its own path through the worst pandemic in 100 years*, Scribe, 2022. Aucante, Yohann. *The Swedish experiment. The Covid-19 response and its controversies*, Bristol University Press, 2022. Sigurd Bergman, and Martin Lindström *Sweden's pandemic experiment*, Routledge, 2022. Czarniawski, Barbara *et al. Covid-19 stories from the Swedish welfare state: The pandemicracy*, Bristol University Press, 2025.

11 Löfven, as note 5, p. 174.

12 Nygren, Katarina Giritli. Anna Olofsson. 'Swedish exceptionalism, herd immunity and the welfare state: A media analysis of struggles over the nature and legitimacy of the Covid-19 pandemic strategy in Sweden', *Sociology, gender studies and cultural studies*, 2021, Vol. 69. No. 4, pp. 529–546, <https://journals.sagepub.com/doi/epub/10.1177/0011392121990025> accessed 18 October 2024.

13 For an examination of Swedish exceptionalism and its decline: Pierre, Jon. 'Introduction: The decline of Swedish exceptionalism?' in Jon Pierre (ed.) *The Oxford Handbook of Swedish politics*, 2016, pp. 1–16.

14 Historical references to Sweden the 'moral superpower' in international relations, hark back to the end of the Second World War, and for more about which see: McKluskey, Emma. 'Viewing noble narratives in security terms: Sweden as poster child of European Integration and integration policy', p. 1., *The Political Studies Association*, <https://www.psa.ac.uk/sites/default/files/767_335.pdf> accessed 17 October 2024.

15 Nygren and Olofsson, as note 12.

16 Baldwin, Peter. 'Sweden stumbles along the third way', in Sigurd Bergman, and Martin Lindström, *Sweden's pandemic experiment*, 2022, p. 1

17 Löfven, Stefan, i samarbete med Ulrika Knutson. *Svetsare och statsminister*, 2024, p. 174.

18 Hansson, Erik *et al.* 'Million-dollar program, migrants, and vulnerability to Covid-19', *Delmi Policy Brief*, 2021:2, <https://migrant-integration.ec.europa.eu/sites/default/files/2021-03/delmi-policy-brief-2021-2.pdf> accessed 7 February 2025.
19 Parkes, Brandon *et al.* 'Community factors and excess mortality in the COVID-19 pandemic in England, Italy and Sweden', p. 697, p. 698, in *European journal of public health*, Vol. 33, No. 4, 2023, pp. 695–703, <https://do.rg/10.1093/eurpub/ckad075> accessed 6 February 2025.
20 Hansson, as note 18.
21 Baldwin, as note 16, p. 1, p. 2, p. 3.
22 Löfven, as note 5, p. 177.
23 Norberg, Johan. 'Sweden during the pandemic. Pariah or paragon?' pp. 10–11, *CATO policy analysis*, No. 959, 29 August 2023, Cato Institute, <https://www.cato.org/sites/cato.org/files/2023-08/policy-analysis-959-no-link.pdf> accessed 6 February 2025.
24 Ibid., p. 10.
25 'Pariah or paragon?' is part of the title of Johan Norberg's article, as note 23.

A Novel Coronavirus – COVID-19

Astrid Lindgren and Pippi, and Sweden

Renowned Swedish fiction writer, Astrid Lindgren (1907–2002), illustrated on the front cover of this book, had been an influential voice in her day, and people listened to what she had to say.

Her writing was to be taken seriously, with a story of hers even leading to changes in Swedish tax law, and towards the end of her long life, Lindgren's influence drew journalists to seek her opinion on anything and everything that had become topical – many of her characters giving credibility to her views.[1] Her most well-known character, Pippi, of *Pippi Longstocking*, who first met Swedish readers in 1945, was principled, defied convention, behaved outside the norm, defiant, and held independent thought.[2]

Had Lindgren been alive in 2020 and experienced the coronavirus pandemic, might she have written a tale for the press on some aspect of COVID-19 in Sweden? Perhaps on the benefit of wearing masks or other face-coverings? Whether she might have or not written a cautionary tale for fellow Swedes, the enduring Pippi was unlikely to have taken the leading role in the story, for traditionally she had exhibited little respect for authority. Nobody would have taken advice from someone defiant of authority seriously enough.

And so, to the real-life story when everything changed around the world, but a little less so in Sweden.

When Everything Changed

Week by week all around the world, the consequences of the COVID-19 pandemic and of the containment and mitigating measures put in place by governments would affect people in different ways, but it was likely to take some time before the effects and influences of the pandemic upon the individual national stories could be assessed or evaluated. It was generally agreed however that they would colour and mark a generation, and its future chances. World economic output had been at least 7 per cent lower than it would otherwise have been, amounting to the biggest slump since the Second World War.[3]

Being a global phenomenon, the pandemic could not be responded to by countries or bodies or agencies in isolation from each other. The virus knew no borders and struck all nations – small or large, and rich or poor – and regardless of politics. As the containment measures – lockdowns – began to be eased in summer 2020, and far too early as it turned out, and as trade flows and supply chains began to be re-established, it was obvious that neither Sweden nor the EU could act on its own. As a global actor, the EU had a responsibility to help frame a global response – through multilateralism and a rules-based international order – with partners in the UN, the WTO, the G20, and the G7, and with countries outside of these intergovernmental political and economic forums.

No matter the subject or science – politics or journalism, history or statistics, political science or public policy, sociology or social policy, economics or finance, epidemiology or virology – COVID-19 and its aftermath was certain to be a focus of research and writing for some years to come. On the everyday and ordinary level, the disease had brought with it new hooks to hang conversation around – one of the first had been 'toilet paper' ('*toapapper*') and why people had been stockpiling it – and it had brought to languages and usage across the world, new concepts, words, and phrases. The range had been wide: 'herd immunity' or '*flockimmunitet*', 'fist bumping' or '*en fist bump*' and 'elbow bumping', 'air hug' and '*luftkram*', 'furlough', 'key worker', 'social distance' and 'physical distance', '*hobbyepidemiologi*' and 'sparetime epidemiology', 'super-spreader' or '*superspridare*', 'lockdown' and 'circuit breaker' (a lesser lockdown) and 'fire-break', 'self-isolation', 'shielding', 'PPE or personal protective equipment', 'test and trace', 'work from home' 'zoom meetings', '*zoom-möten*' , 'R-numbers' and 'infection rates', 'new normal', 'pandemic', 'self-quarantine' or '*självkarantän*', 'travel bubbles' and 'support bubbles', 'travel corridors' and 'air bridges', 'hotspots', 'long-COVID' or 'post-COVID-19 condition' (PCC), the 'Great Barrington Declaration', the 'John Snow Memorandum', 'the 22 researchers', 'mutations' and 'variants of the virus', 'vaccine nationalism', 'vaccination passports', '*gröna beviset*' or 'the green digital certificate', getting 'pinged' or '*pingade*' to start self-isolation, and 'pingdemic' or '*pingdemi*'. Would these be part of language long-term, or would they drop away, proving to be ephemeral as the pandemic gave way to an endemic COVID-19? Would they be found in tomorrow's dictionaries, encyclopaedias, or online reference works?

Inarguable was the fact that the pandemic had swept away old political agendas, and that the national and global crises brought in its wake would fundamentally change societies and politics and those of every other country in the world, also for many years to come. An exaggeration perhaps, but at the very least coronavirus had certainly given Sweden's right-wing and populist Sweden Democrats much less opportunity to talk about immigration and crime. Abroad, media talk was all about Sweden's strategy to fight the virus.

During the early months of 2020 the world's media bore down on Sweden for the seemingly unique approach taken by public health authorities and the government in handling the COVID-19 crisis. The spotlight gave Sweden a high international profile, shining down hard on its society, and on its prime minister Stefan Löfven (in post 2014–22). Also under the glare were health and social affairs minister Lena Hallengren, the recently appointed foreign minister Ann Linde and her team, Olivia Wigzell of the board of health and welfare, and the country's epidemiologists and virologists, not least Anders Tegnell the chief epidemiologist at the public health agency, and Johan Carlson director-general of the agency. Funding the country's mitigation measures had been the remit of finance minister Magdalena Andersson (in post since 2014, and subsequently Sweden's first female prime minister, 2021–22). Over time, all would joke that they had seen much more of each other than of their families.[4]

Arrival of the Virus – Counterattack Begins From the Very Start – 'Next Generation EU'

At the close of December 2019, the WHO China Country Office had been informed of a pneumonia-like illness of unknown cause that had gripped the Hubei Province of China.[5] A novel coronavirus outbreak – a severe acute respiratory syndrome-related coronavirus – had emerged.

On 12 January 2020, China shared publicly the genetic sequence of the novel coronavirus which became provisionally named 2019-nCoV by the Coronaviridae Study Group (CSG) of the International Committee on Taxonomy of Viruses (ICTV). As a close relative, or sister clade (having an immediate common ancestor), to the prototype human and bat severe acute respiratory syndrome-related (SARS) coronaviruses, it was subsequently designated as SARS-CoV-2.[6]

There were hundreds of coronaviruses, most of them circulating among animals such as pigs, camels, bats, and cats (more than sixty mammal species alone), but which sometimes jumped to humans. Four of the seven coronaviruses known in 2020 to cause sickness among humans caused only mild to moderate disease, but three could cause more serious and fatal disease. An earlier SARS-CoV (SARS coronavirus) which emerged in 2002 – possibly originating in bats, a reservoir for SARS-like coronaviruses – had infected more than 8,000 people and killed 774. Middle East respiratory syndrome (MERS) identified in 2012 was caused by the MERS coronavirus, MERS-CoV, transmitted from camels. Now SARS-CoV-2 had emerged.[7] In 2016–17, a novel coronavirus identified among piglets in Guangdong Province in China had emerged from the same bat species causing SARS-CoV and was named swine acute diarrhoea syndrome (SADS) coronavirus, or SADS-CoV.[8] In March 2021, the final report of a global study into the origins of SARS-CoV-2 which had been conducted by the WHO in Wuhan – focussing in particular on the Huanan Seafood Wholesale Market – found that the most likely pathway into the human population had been through direct zoonotic spillover, from bats, and that introduction through an intermediate animal host was also to considered likely.[9]

The identification and sharing of the genetic sequence of the coronavirus had been the starting gun for a counterattack by vaccine scientists – virologists, bacteriologists, immunologists, microbiologists, and epidemiologists – who had been preparing for years for just such a virus. Around the world they sprang into action, working in different ways to turn the virus into candidate vaccines to fight the pandemic, and several were in the vanguard. The Chinese Centre for Disease Control, and Prevention (CCDC), working with state-owned, but separate, pharmaceutical partners Sinopharm and Sinovac, began developing inactivated virus vaccines (using the whole virus to trigger an immune response). In the USA, at the National Institutes of Health (NIH), mRNA vaccine was being worked on (using genetic material to provide cells with the instructions to make the antigen). Pfizer Inc., a multinational pharmaceutical and biotechnology company in the USA, together with BioNTech SE in Germany, were also working on mRNA vaccines. In the UK, Oxford University together with AstraZeneca, a UK-Swedish multinational pharmaceutical and biotechnology firm, began work on a vector vaccine (using a harmless virus as the carrier to deliver instructions to the cell). The Gamaleya Research Institute of Epidemiology and Microbiology in Russia (the Gam-COVID-Vac, or Sputnik V vaccine) also began work on a vector vaccine, as did Janssen Pharmaceuticals (Johnson & Johnson) in the Netherlands and Belgium. In Australia, the University of Queensland working with CSL Ltd. focussed on the development of a protein or subunit vaccine (using a very specific part of the virus that the immune system needed to recognize, and in this case adding a fragment of protein found on the HIV virus). Novavax Inc. of Maryland, USA, also began work on a protein vaccine. Most of these candidate vaccines went on to successful clinical trial outside their respective laboratories and to become well-known COVID-19 vaccines, but one dropped by the wayside – the protein vaccine candidate worked on by University of Queensland/CSL).[10]

Meanwhile, just as the starting gun for the counterattack had been fired, and just as the Chinese New Year Festivals got into full swing between 17 January and 8 February – Little Year, Spring Festival and Lantern Festival – with 400 million Chinese travelling across the vast country, including 7 million travelling abroad, cases of the virus (SARS-CoV-2) were being reported in South Korea, Japan, Thailand, and Singapore. On 30 January 2020, the WHO had declared the outbreak as a Public Health Emergency of International Concern (PHEIC).[11]

On 28 January, the Croatian presidency of the Council of the EU (January–June 2020) activated the EU's Integrated Political Crisis Response (IPCR) arrangements to information sharing mode. This move triggered the production of integrated reports by the EU Commission and the European External Action Service (EEAS) – the EU's diplomatic service and combined foreign and defence ministry – and the creation of a dedicated page on the IPCR web platform on which information about the outbreak was shared.[12] Europe was getting itself ready.

On 11 February, SARS-CoV-2 was named COVID-19, a name chosen within WHO guidelines which required that it be pronounceable and non-stigmatizing, and that it did not refer to a geographical location, an animal, an individual or group of people.[13] Nevertheless, throughout 2020 and into 2021, news organisations and even governments would refer to new coronavirus variants by the country in which they were first identified (and it would not be until May 2021 before the WHO announced geographically and politically neutral Greek letter names for new variants – Alpha, Beta, and so on).

In February, EU health ministers exchanged views on the implications of the outbreak, discussing measures and activities being undertaken and how to strengthen cooperation in areas of public health.[14]

At the end of February, Italy had reported a significant increase of COVID-19 cases concentrated in its northern regions and most other EU member states had started reporting cases of the disease.[15]

Into March, health authorities in Italy and Iran had begun to be stretched by the outbreak, and at a media briefing on 11 March, Dr Tedros Adhanom Ghebreyesus, director-general of the WHO, formally characterised COVID-19 as a global pandemic. Also on 11 March, by video conference, members of the European Council discussed how to coordinate EU efforts to respond to COVID-19, covering areas such as limiting the spread of the virus, the provision of medical equipment particularly masks and respirators, promoting research including research into a vaccine, and tackling the socio-economic consequences of the disease.[16]

On 26 March, heads of government participating in a European Council summit (by video conference) had called for a coordinated exit strategy from the lockdown measures – of varying degrees – that had been put in place, as well as a comprehensive recovery plan and unprecedented investment. In consultation with other institutions, particularly the European Central Bank (ECB), the president of the European Council and the president of the EU Commission were invited to start work on a roadmap towards a recovery plan.[17]

On 23 April, Charles Michel, president of the European Council, and other members of the Council participated in a video conference tasked to give the go-ahead to a safety net from the Eurogroup of EUR 540 billion, and to reach agreement on a European recovery fund.[18]

On 27 May, and arising out of the video conference, the Commission published its proposal for a recovery fund and an updated EU long-term budget – the Multiannual Financial Framework, MFF – for 2021–27. While the title *EU budget powering the recovery plan for Europe* was a descriptive but rather mundane one for the proposal, the content described the creation of a new recovery instrument, 'Next Generation EU'. Using its strong triple-A credit rating, the Commission would borrow EUR 750 billion (SEK 7,800 billion) on the financial markets to be repaid over a long period and throughout future EU budgets, between 2028 and 2058. To meet the most pressing needs, the current MFF for 2014–20 would be amended to make EUR 11.5 billion available for immediate funding. The EUR 750 billion raised on the markets for 'Next Generation EU' would be invested across three pillars: supporting member states with investments and reforms; kick-starting the EU economy by incentivising private investment; and addressing the lessons of the pandemic crisis.[19]

Support to member states was to include a new recovery and resilience facility which would offer financial support for investment and reforms, including green transition and digital transformation, and although open to all members it would be concentrated on the most affected and where resilience needs were greatest.[20] Though grumbles from Poland and Hungary were exposed by the recovery package, agreement had been reached – a provisional agreement at least – by the end of the year and the meeting of the European Council, 10–11 December 2020.

Back in March too had come the call from G20 leaders for a global response to the pandemic, and in an answer to that call, the WHO, the EU Commission, the Bill and Melinda Gates Foundation (with the Global Alliance for Vaccines and Immunizations, GAVI) and France, had co-launched in April the Access to COVID-19 Tools Accelerator (ACT-A). This would be a global collaboration bringing together governments, global health organisations, manufacturers, scientists, the private sector, civil society and philanthropy to provide innovative and equitable access to COVID-19 diagnostics, treatment, and vaccines. ACT-A and its COVAX facility would speed up the search for effective vaccines and equitable access to them for all countries.[21]

Swedish Time-Line – Mitigation Measures Taken – Löfven, Address to the Nation, March 2020 – Eurovision 2020

Testing the resources of every country in the world, the virus had been confirmed in Sweden for the first time in Jönköping in late-January 2020, though there may have been cases in the country as early as November 2019.

There had been reports of foreign participants in the 2019 Military World Games held in Wuhan in late-October having fallen sick. These included some armed forces personnel and family members from Sweden's Norrbotten Regiment (*Norbottens regementet, I19*, garrisoned at Boden) who had felt coronavirus symptoms both while they were in China and after their return. Those affected by the flu-like symptoms were described by the regimental doctor as having been in the 20–45 age bracket and physically well-trained. While some were back in post after a week, others were unable to resume training until after a month. None had tested positive for COVID-19. Personnel at another unit in southern Sweden also had reported odd symptoms after the visit to China. Published in 2021, an Irish study found there was indeed a correlation between the number of individuals who travelled to the 2019 Games and the number of COVID-19 cases in the country to which attendees returned. Whether that explained the rapid spread of the pandemic or not was not known definitively.[22]

On 1 February, the Swedish government classified COVID-19 as a disease that constituted a danger to society, opening the possibility of extraordinary communicable disease control measures. Well into February cases began to be reported among individuals who had been on holiday in Italy

From early-March, anyone in the country with symptoms of respiratory infection, even if only mild ones, was urged to avoid social contact both within the workplace and in private spheres. On 11 March, the day that the WHO declared the outbreak to be a global pandemic, Sweden's first recorded death from COVID-19 occurred at the Karolinska University Hospital (*Karolinska Universitetssjukhuset*) one of Europe's premier health facilities in Huddinge, Stockholm, the largest hospital in the region (affiliated to the Karolinska Institute, one of Sweden's oldest medical schools). The victim who had been over 70 years old with underlying health problems had contracted the disease through community transmission. On 16 March, Sweden's public health agency (*Folkhälsomyndigheten*) recommended isolating people over seventy and recommended working from home.[23]

Meanwhile, Sweden had begun scaling up the number of intensive care beds, with the Karolinska increasing its capacity significantly. At the start of the crisis, Sweden was estimated to have just over 500 intensive care beds, which was 5.8 intensive care beds per 100,000 people, compared to a European average of 11.5.

In just a matter of weeks 1,100 beds were available – a doubling of capacity – with the Karolinska increasing from thirty-eight intensive care beds to 200.[24]

In an effort to mitigate the effects of the outbreak of the COVID-19 virus and to reduce its spread, in mid-March, the foreign affairs ministry had advised against non-essential travel to all countries, and on 17 March – in response to the call from the European Council and the European Commission – the government placed a temporary stop, a ban, on non-essential travel into Sweden as well, except from countries in the EEA, and from Switzerland and the UK. Swedish citizens were not affected by the entry ban, nor did it prevent travel within the EU.[25] As the crisis developed however, members states did begin to close their borders on each other.

By 18 March, many upper secondary schools – students aged sixteen and over – and all universities had switched over to distance learning. Schools for younger children, lower secondary and primary schools and kindergartens remained open. The government had wanted to keep Sweden open as much as possible – did not want to close society down – and advised that lockdown would bring loneliness and resulting mental problems, doubly affecting children not allowed to go to school. If schools had been closed, teachers, doctors, nurses, and bus drivers would be forced to stay at home and look after their children. That would hasten a lockdown, which said Löfven 'we wanted to avoid as long as we could'. Production would have stopped, and the economy damaged, if people had stayed at home, away from the workplace. Schools would be the last thing to close, and the first to reopen.[26]

Of importance for the future was the question of learning loss when students were not allowed to go to school for months on end.

Although schools had been kept open, events that might encourage more than fifty persons were banned from 27 March, pubs and restaurants served only seated customers (table service), relatives were told to avoid unnecessary visits to hospital, and from 1 April a ban on visiting elderly care institutions (*ålderdomshem*) was imposed.[27]

Earlier, on 22 March, Löfven, had addressed the nation, stating that coronavirus was 'testing our country, our society and us as human beings' and that the next few months would 'be stressful'. We would 'face the crisis as a society'. Following the advice of the public health authorities was the duty of every person, 'yours – and mine'. We all had 'a great responsibility'. The aim, he said, was to limit the spread of infection, so that a lot of people would not be ill at the same time. He asked Swedes to be prepared for the fact that this would 'last for a long time' and to be 'ready for the situation changing quickly'. While the restrictions might be stressful, it was through these that the healthcare system would be able to handle the crisis. There would be, he said, a few crucial moments in life when we had 'to make sacrifices' for those around us, for our fellow human beings, 'and for our country'. Adding gravity and statesmanship to his address, 'That moment is now. That day is here', he said, and the task applied to everyone.[28]

It had been rare for a prime minister to give a speech to the nation, though he had done it once before after a terrorist outrage in central Stockholm in 2017, an attack in the busy and popular shopping street, Drottninggatan, when a hijacked truck was driven into crowds and then crashed into the corner of Åhléns City department store. Prior to that, former prime minister Göran Persson had spoken to the nation after the murder of foreign minister Anna Lindh in 2003 in the Nordiska Kompaniet (NK) department store in central Stockholm.[29] Löfven's prime ministerial speech had come a few days after the pandemic had claimed its first Swedish victim, and later, in his autobiography, he wrote 'we understood that over time there could be many more deaths'. His address had brought common purpose, and a cooling down of political arguments and debates around employment law, migration policy, violence, and crime.

As the crisis had developed, information given to Swedes from the public health agency and local health authorities had differed little from that offered to the citizens of other EU countries. In brief, the advice was to: stay at home if any cold- or flu-like symptoms developed; practice good hygiene by, for example, washing hands for at least 20 seconds with soap and warm water; keep distance from people when in public places; avoid large gatherings and limit social contacts; work from home if able to; avoid using forms of public transport where tickets could not be booked; avoid public transport at busy times; and, if over 70 years old, or belonging to a high-risk group, stay at home and reduce all social contacts.[30]

In the approach to limiting the spread of infection – containment strategy – the government was in charge (in a whole-of-government approach), but expert national agencies and international bodies would play a key role. The strategy had several intended actions: to ensure healthcare resources were available; to limit the impact of the disease on critical services; to alleviate the impact on people and companies; to ease concerns by, for example, providing information; and, to ensure that the right measures were taken at the right time, with flexible adjustment to developments on the ground. A top priority was the protection of the elderly and the vulnerable, and another was the fostering of public trust.[31]

The overall objective was to reduce the pace of spread of the virus – to 'flatten the curve' became the widely used expression – so that large numbers of people did not become ill at the same time. The measures taken to reduce the pace of spread needed to be weighed against their effects on society and public health in general, and an important starting point in taking measures was careful consideration of the knowledge of experts. Swedes had a high level of trust in government agencies, and this meant that a large proportion of them followed the advice given.[32]

To mitigate the financial impact of the pandemic on Swedish businesses, organisations, and agencies, and to save people's jobs and livings, the government presented comprehensive crisis packages and fiscal measures to support municipalities and regions, individuals and companies and businesses. The OECD estimated the packages at some SEK 661.8 billion (around EUR 62.1 billion) which was nearly 13 per cent of GDP.[33]

Central government planned to compensate municipalities and regions for putting in place extraordinary measures and extra costs in health and medical care associated with the COVID-19 virus. On 2 April this was placed at SEK 3 billion, a rise from an earlier SEK 2 billion. Additionally, grants to municipalities and regions would increase by SEK 20 billion in 2020, a rise from a previously planned SEK 5 billion. Sickness benefit was to be paid from the first day of illness and the government would assume the entire cost of all sick pay during April and May 2020.[34]

From 1 May, and for three months, employers would be able to reduce employee working hours by up to 80 per cent and the government would bear most of the cost. Wage costs would be reduced by over 70 per cent, while employees would retain almost 90 per cent of their original wage. There would be a temporary reduction in employer's social security contributions to the old age pension contribution for the period 1 March to 30 June 2020 only. For sole proprietors of small businesses, VAT reported annually from December 2019 to January 2021 would be eligible for deferral.[35]

There would also be support amounting to SEK 500 million for cultural activities losing revenue as a result of restrictions on public events, and the same amount for sports.[36]

While much of the world had gone into lockdown – either advised by governments or imposed by governments – Sweden appeared to have taken a radically different approach. Although social life had become centred on the home, and distancing measures were being taken when outside of it – as it had done elsewhere in Europe – Sweden kept businesses, offices, shops, primary schools and nurseries open albeit with some restrictions. Enclosed spaces were being avoided however, and on Stockholm's public transport network commuters kept distance from each other. Additionally, trips away to popular Swedish resorts such as Åre, or Sälen, or Idre Fjäll planned for the annual school winter sports holiday (*sportlov*) – falling in late-February and early-March – had been cancelled or cut short.[37] Also curtailed were the Valborg revelries held over 30 April into 1 May (*Valborgsmässoafton* or *Walpurgisnacht*) particularly popular in the smaller and older student cities such as Lund and Uppsala, and which required bonfires, song, fireworks and refreshment as an offering to spring. Due to the ban on public events attracting more than fifty people, Valborg 2020 would be a quieter affair with bonfires and fireworks livestreamed and public parks scattered with chicken manure to deter people from gathering. Traditional means of marking May Day itself – demonstrations and marches by the Social Democrats and Left Party – would also be cancelled.[38]

Another casualty of COVID-19 had been the 2020 Eurovision Song Contest, one of those events that marked the course of the year, and which had been scheduled to take place in Rotterdam on 16 May. While Eurovision organizers had explored many alternative options to staging the show, the banning of large public gatherings by the Dutch government, the uncertainties created by the spread of coronavirus, and international travel restrictions, meant cancellation had been the only option, difficult though that decision had been. Sweden was to have been represented in Rotterdam by 'The Mamas', winners of the annual *Melodifestival*, the national selection competition for Eurovision. Formal cancellation of Eurovision 2020 by the European Broadcasting Union (EBU) had been announced on 18 March, the same day that the cancellation of the Glastonbury Festival in England had been announced.[39]

Chapter 2 will consider criticism of the high-risk Swedish approach to COVID-19, and defence of the strategy. What were the criticisms that had been put forward? What role had public trust in science, government, and authorities played in the Swedish approach to the pandemic?

Notes

1 'Astrid Lindgren – a voice to be reckoned with. Writing *Pippi Longstocking* made her famous, but did you know that Astrid Lindgren was also an opinion former?' Sweden.se, <https://sweden.se/life/people/astrid-lindgren-a-voice-to-be-reckoned-with> accessed 5 February 2025. The story that had changed Swedish tax law was *Pomperipossa in Monismania* (March 1976), an opinion piece (*debatartikel*) published by the tabloid *Expressen* highlighting the level of income tax the self-employed Lindgren had to pay.

2 Schlessinger, June H. 'Pippi Longstocking by Astrid Lindgren', Research Starters Home, EBSCO, 2022, <https://www.ebsco.com/research-starters/literature-and-writing/pippi-longstocking-astrid-lindgren#context> accessed 24 April 2025, and Haager, Julia Sophie. 'What makes Pippi Longstocking a classic of identity empowerment?' Programme Research, *Televizion*, 29/2016/E, 22 May 2016, <https://izi.br.de/english/publication/televizion/20_2016_E/Haager-What_makes_Pippi_Longstocking_a_classic.pdf> accessed 20 May 2025.

3 'The plague year', *The Economist*, Vol. 437, No. 9225, 19 December 2020, p. 17.

4 Löfven, Stefan. i samarbete med Ulrika Knutson. *Svetsare och statsminister*, 2024, p. 172.

5 'Rolling updates on coronavirus disease (COVID-19)', World Health Organization (WHO), <https://www.who.int/emergencies/diseases/novel-coronavirus-2019/events-as-they-happen> accessed 5 June 2019.

6 'The species Severe acute respiratory syndrome-related coronavirus: classifying 2019- nCoV and naming it SARS-CoV-2', *Nature Microbiology*, 5, pp. 536–44, 2 March 2020, <https://doi.org/10.1038/s41564-020-0695-z> accessed 27 June 2020.

7 'Coronaviruses', National Institute of Allergy and Infectious Diseases (NIAID), National Institutes of Health (NIH), <https://www.niaid.nih.gov/diseases-conditions/coronaviruses> accessed 12 October 2020.

8 'New coronavirus emerges from bats in China, devastates young swine', National Institutes of Health (NIH), 4 April 2018, <https://www.nih.gov/news-events/news-releases/new-coronavirus-emerges-bats-china-devastates-young-swine> accessed 12 October 2020.

9 'WHO-convened Global Study of Origins of SARS-CoV-2: China Part', Joint WHO-China Study 14 January-10 February 2021, Joint Report, WHO, p. 8, <https://www.who.int/publications/i/item/who-convened-global-study-of-origins-of-sars-cov-2-china-part> accessed 30 March 2021. Zoonotic spillover is the spread of germs between animals and people. COVID-19 is a zoonotic disease.

10 *The Vaccine—A Horizon Special*, Horizon, BBC 2, Tuesday, 22 June 2021 (Wingspan Productions, and Global Health Reporting Center, in collaboration with HHMI/Tangled Bank Studios, for BBC/CNN Film. 2021, and with producer/director, Catherine Gale).

11 World Health Organization, as note 5.

12 'COVID-19 outbreak: the presidency steps up EU response by triggering full activation mode of IPCR', Press release, European Council / Council of the European Union, 2 March 2020, <https://www.consilium.europa.eu/en/press/press-releases/2020/03/02/covid-19-outbreak-the-presidency-steps-up-eu-response-by-triggering-full-activation-mode-of-ipcr/> accessed 20 July 2020.

13 World Health Organization, as note 5.

14 'Employment, Social Policy, Health and Consumer Affairs Council (Health'), Meetings, European Council / Council of the European Union', 13 February 2020, <https://www.consilium.europa.eu/en/meetings/epsco/2020/02/13/> accessed 20 July 2020.

15 'COVID-19 coronavirus pandemic', European Council / Council of the European Union, <https://www.consilium.europa.eu/en/policies/coronavirus> accessed 20 July 2020.

16 World Health Organization, as note 5, and, Video conference of the members of the European Council, 10 March 2020, European Council / Council of the European Union, <https://www.consilium.europa.eu/en/meetings/european-council/2020/03/10/> accessed 20 July 2020.

17 'A roadmap for recovery. Towards a more resilient, sustainable and fair Europe', European Council / Council of the European Union, 21 April 2020, p. 1, <https://www.consilium.europa.eu/media/43384/roadmap-for-recovery-final-21-04-2020.pdf> accessed 20 July 2020.

18 'Conclusions of the President of the European Council following the video conference of the members of the European Council, 23 April 2020', European Council / Council of the European Union, 23 April 2020, <https://www.consilium.europa.eu/en/press/press-releases/2020/04/23/conclusions-by-president-charles-michel-following-the-video-conference-with-members-of-the-european-council-on-23-april-2020/> accessed 21 July 2020.

19 'Europe's moment: Repair and prepare for the next generation', Press release, European Commission, 27 May 2020, <https://ec.europa.eu/commission/presscorner/detail/en/p_20_940> accessed 21 July 2020.

20 Ibid.

21 'Covax: Working for global equitable access to Covid-19 vaccines', World Health Organization (WHO), <https://www.who.int/initiatives/act-accelerator/covax> accessed 15 December 2020.

22 'Regementsläkaren: åtta norrbottningar har provtagits', *Norrländska Socialdemokraten NSD*, 15 April 2020, <https://nsd.se/nyheter/regementslakaren-atta-norrbottningar-har-provtagits-nm5340524.aspx> accessed 12 June 2020, and, Winter, Amy Elise. 'The impact of the World Military Games on the Covid-19 pandemic', *Irish journal of medical science*, 190 (4), 19 January 2021, pp. 1653–1654, <https://doi.org/10.1007/s11845-020-02484-0> accessed 16 May 2025.

23 'Tackling coronavirus (COVID-19). Contributing to a global effort. Sweden. Containment measures', OECD, 15 April 2020, <http://www.oecd.org/coronavirus/en/> accessed 26 April 2020. The Karolinska Institute is named after Karl XIII who founded it in 1810 for the training of army field-surgeons.

24 Löfgren, Emma. 'The biggest challenge of our time: How Sweden doubled intensive care capacity amid COVID-19 panic', *The Local*, 23 June 2020, <https://www.thelocal.se/20200623/how-sweden-doubled-intensive-care-capacity-to-treat-coronavirus-patients> accessed 29 June 2020.

25 OECD, as note 20.

26 Löfven, as note 4, pp.173–4, p. 179.

27 OECD, as note 20.

28 'Prime Minister Stefan Löfven's address to the nation' /' Statsminister Stefan Lövens tal till nationen', Government Offices of Sweden, Stockholm, 22 March 2020, <https://www.regeringen.se/tal/2020/03/statsministerns-tal-till-nationen-den-22-mars-2020/> accessed 26 April 2020.

29 Löfven, as note 4, p. 172

30 'Coronavirus: These are the official recommendations you should still be following in Sweden', *The Local*, 28 February 2020, and updated, <https://www.thelocal.se/20200228/coronavirus-the-everyday-precautions-to-take-if-you-are-in-Sweden> accessed 3 July 2020.

31 'Sweden's response to COVID-19', PowerPoint presentation, Ministry for Health and Social Affairs, Government Offices of Sweden, Stockholm, <https://www.government.se/49960e/globalassets/government/dokument/socialdepartementet/powerpoint-presentation-sweden-ministry-of-health-23-april-who-briefing-pdf.pdf> and, 'The government's work in response to the virus responsible for COVID-19', Government Offices of Sweden. Stockholm, <https://www.government.se/government-policy/the-governments-work-in-response-to-the-virus-responsible-for-covid-19/?page=7> accessed 12 June 2020.

32 'Strategy in response to the COVID-19 pandemic', Government Offices of Sweden, Stockholm, 6 April 2020, <https://www.government.se/articles/2020/04/strategy-in-response-to-the-covid-19-pandemic/> accessed 26 April 2020.

33 OECD, as note 20.

34 Ibid.

35 Ibid.

36 Ibid.

37 Pancevski, Bojan. and Dominic Chopping. 'Inside Sweden's radically different approach to the coronavirus', *The Wall Street Journal*, 30 March 2020. <https://www.wsj.com/articles/inside-swedens-radically-different-approach-to-the-coronavirus-11585598175> accessed 26 April 2020.

38 'How the coronavirus is changing one of Sweden's most famous holidays', *The Local*, 29 April 2020, <https://thelocal.se/20200529/how-the-coronavirus-has-changed-walpurgis-and-may-day-celebrations-in-sweden> accessed 12 June 2020.

39 'Eurovision Song Contest 2020 cancelled', EBU, <https://www.ebu.ch/news/2020/03/eurovision-song-contest-2020-cancelled> accessed 16 May 2025.

Criticism and Defence

Domestic Criticism – HighRisk Strategy

Anders Tegnell, chief epidemiologist at the public health agency, had said that the overall objective of reducing the pace of spread of the virus – flattening the curve – and at the same time sheltering the elderly and the vulnerable until a vaccine became available, would also bring a natural immunity among the population.[1]

Allowing the virus to propagate through the population in this controlled manner in order to build a natural form of immunity – developing herd immunity – had also been briefly considered by the UK and the Netherlands, but after scientists warned they could face hundreds of thousands of deaths and an overwhelmed healthcare system each had reversed their decisions.[2]

The Swedish approach was not without criticism at home, and anxieties had been raised by scientists and doctors themselves early on, some concerned that COVID-19 cases would pick up fast. In mid-March, Joacim Rocklöv, a professor of epidemiology at Umeå University, said that the Swedish approach was highrisk and that it could have catastrophic consequences. COVID-19 was a serious disease, and Sweden was no different from other countries. The pursuit of herd immunity without suppressing the spread of the virus would overwhelm hospitals and result in large numbers of premature deaths. He was also sceptical that vulnerable groups could be effectively sheltered.[3] Sweden needed 'tough measures' Rocklöv said, otherwise the healthcare system would have to prioritize some of its intensive care patients over others – would have to make choices as to who had the best chance of survival – as had happened in Italy.[4]

Also based at Umeå University, Fredrik Elgh, a professor of virology, had said that Swedish policy was frightening and called for Stockholm to be put under quarantine, otherwise cases would overwhelm the system further down the epidemic curve. At the same time though, some European experts and officials, including the prominent German doctor, Ansgar Lohse, at the University

Medical Centre Hamburg-Eppendorf (UKE), and Sir Patrick Vallance, chief scientific adviser to the British government, had praised the approach, joining experts who had said that the only way to curb the epidemic before the emergence of a vaccine was to gradually create herd immunity.[5]

In August, freelance journalist Emanuel Karlsten would reveal internal emails from mid-March showing discussions on herd immunity between Tegnell and the former state epidemiologist Johan Giesecke, and exchanges with Mika Salminen, Tegnell's counterpart in Finland. One email forwarded to Salminen had suggested allowing healthy people to get infected voluntarily and in controlled settings, and that schools might be kept open to reach herd immunity more quickly. The R-rate or R-number – the R0 or basic reproduction number, a measure of the infection rate which ideally should be kept below 1 – had also been discussed between Tegnell and Giesecke. The email exchanges, Karlsten suggested, showed a sort of brainstorming between colleagues and that even in retirement, Giesecke continued to hold significant influence.[6] That latter point – keeping schools open – would prove interesting, as testing in Sweden was showing a low spread of infection among children and teenagers.

Karlsten's revelations had been posted on his own blog after submitting freedom of information requests to the public health agency and to the Karolinska Institute where Giesecke was professor emeritus. In a more sensationalist article in *Expressen*, Karlsten highlighted an email from Geisecke to a Swedish pension fund in mid-March in which he said that COVID-19 would sweep like a storm over Sweden, infecting everyone in one or two months. He believed that thousands were already infected in Sweden and that it would all end when so many had been infected and become immune that the virus would have nowhere else to go (in other words, when Sweden had achieved herd immunity).[7] Giesecke, it would later show, had been very wide of the mark, with Sweden having reached only very low levels of immunity by May.

Foreign Criticism – Sweden an Experiment

The view abroad was that life in Sweden had been carrying on as normal and that a strategy based on pursuing herd immunity – accepting a scale of infection across the population enough to prevent further spread – was endangering too many people in the interests of the economy.[8]

Sweden had been described as an 'outrider' by some – in the vanguard by others – and an experiment being followed closely by other countries. There had been no lockdown, just light touch regulation, with citizens 'expected to keep a safe distance' and 'not ordered to stay home'.[9] Sweden was an 'outlier' – lying well outside the normal range of behaviour.[10]

Defending the Strategy

While herd immunity had indeed been talked of as a possible side effect of the strategy, it was not the primary aim. The aim had been to limit the spread of the disease while avoiding some of the worst of the social, economic, and medical consequences of the pandemic.[11]

In a Sunday morning BBC television conversation with Isabella Lövin, Green politician and minister for environment and climate and deputy prime minister in the Löfven cabinet, journalist Andrew Marr had raised the issue of herd immunity. He quoted Tegnell as having said that Stockholm was quite close to achieving herd immunity and that all of Sweden was not far behind, and he asked the minister if herd immunity was part of the Swedish strategy. This had not been the case, Lövin said, rather the strategy had been to confine the spread of the virus and limit deaths and cases of the disease in the population. And besides, she said, there was no way of knowing as yet when an individual had achieved immunity.[12]

Sweden's approach was based on scientific advice and a two-way trust: a population trusting in the strategy being taken, trust in the government, and trust of authorities and agencies in the ability of citizens to act responsibly. And there was a societal basis to that trust: a level playing field with most people enjoying the same basic education and healthcare, and a long tradition of trusting in science.[13]

Trust had been an issue raised by Marr in his conversation with Lövin when he remarked that the Swedish population was by-and-large trusting of its government and was doing as it was asked to do. He asked how important it was to the building of trust that there be transparent and open communication from the government. This was crucial answered the minister, open communication was fundamental to building trust between the government and people. Government needed to be as transparent as possible. Along with trust came great responsibility, and it was the responsibility of everyone to listen to what the experts were saying – real experts and not who Löfven had described as '*hobbyepidemiologier*' ('sparetime epidemiologists').[14] Sceptical BBC viewers would doubtless make comparisons between Sweden and the UK on the matter of trust, responsibility, and listening to experts, always with the controversial figure of Boris Johnson at the back of their minds.

Lövin said that every had country had set out to limit the spread of the virus, and Sweden was no exception. They had realized from the very start that countering the virus, and the effort required, was not going to be a sprint but a marathon. It would be wrong, she said – a great myth – to say that the steps Sweden had taken to address the pandemic had not really been serious.[15]

Picking up on the comment that the effort was going to be a marathon rather than a sprint, and that it was still early in the story, Marr had asked if Sweden was warning other countries that had imposed higher levels of lockdown – such as the UK – that in the end there might be some kind of reaction to these, and that overall it might have been better to have been more relaxed from the start. The minister had responded by saying that every country needed to impose measures that were in accordance with its own traditions and system of governance,[16] and of course here she was alluding to the exercising of 'collective decision-making' in the Swedish government system, and the prohibition on 'ministerial rule'. No individual minister had the power to intervene directly in a decision taken in the day-to-day running of a government agency (the public health agency for Sweden for example) or in a specific matter relating to the due exercise of the agency's authority.[17]

Long-Term Strategy

Measures that were too harsh, Lövin said, could not be sustained over a long period of time. There might be a reaction to them, with people no longer respecting the voluntary recommendations – the 'general recommendations' or *allmänna råd* – that really needed to be respected over an extended period (the marathon), and until a vaccine was found. The government did not want to fatigue the people when they were largely supportive of a strategy which had not come without impact on the economy, freedoms, and employment.[18]

Tegnell believed that Sweden would be able to sustain its own version of the 'new normal' for an extended period. Those countries that had imposed tough and controlled lockdowns would have to end them sooner or later, facing the possibility of caseloads spiralling upwards again, out of control.[19] Nevertheless, in countries that had imposed strict lockdowns (France, Italy), the strategy had proved to be effective with death rates dropping drastically. In New Zealand which had pre-empted a large-scale outbreak with an early lockdown, the virus appeared to have been almost eliminated by the end of May 2020. In Sweden, where there had been a lack of lockdown, the infection rate showed no sign of falling.[20]

In addition, by May, Sweden had been nowhere near the threshold needed for herd immunity – that possible side effect of its strategy. Scientists had suggested that 60 per cent of a population would need to have COVID-19 antibodies before herd immunity was reached. The Swedish government had hoped for 20 per cent by the end of May, but only 7.3 per cent had them.[21]

Chapter 3 will look at the Swedish death rate and R-rate during the peak months of the crisis, as well as social and cultural differences affecting the death rate. How wide of the mark had been the modelling and warnings from foreign critics that Sweden would have 100,000 deaths by June 2020? Why had Sweden such a high death toll in comparison to the rest of Scandinavia? Why was the virus hitting hardest the immigrant communities in Stockholm's suburbs? Had the differing multigenerational interactions within migrant families compared to a non-migrant families played a role in spreading the virus to the elderly?

Notes

1 Pancevski, Bojan. and Dominic Chopping. 'Inside Sweden's radically different approach to the coronavirus', *The Wall Street Journal*, 30 March 2020. <https://www.wsj.com/articles/inside-swedens-radically-different-approach-to-the-coronavirus-11585598175> accessed 26 April 2020.

2 Ibid.

3 Ibid.

4 Holm, Gusten. 'Professorn: Sverige kan få Italiens situation', *Expressen*, 15 March 2020, <https://www.expressen.se/nyheter/professorn-sverige-kanfa-italiens-situation/> accessed 4 June 2020.

5 Pancevski, as note 1, and, Pancevski, Bojan. 'German infectiologist Ansgar Lohse joins experts who say [...]' [Twitter post] @bopanc, 29 March 2020, <https://twitter.com/bopanc/status/1244285493107478535?lang=en> accessed 4 June 2020.

6 Karlsten, Emanuel. 'Tegnell-mejlen: Så fick flockimmuniteten fäste hos Folkhälsomyndigheten', Emanuel Karlsten website, 12 August 2020, <https://emanuelkarlsten.se/tegnell-mejlen-sa-fick-flockimmuniteten-faste-hos-folkhalsomyndigheten/> and, Orange, Richard. 'Why is everyone in Sweden talking about Anders Tegnell's emails?' *The Local*, 12 August 2020, <https://www.thelocal.se/20200812/why-is-everyone-taking-about-anders-tegnells-emails> accessed 15 August 2020.

7 Karlsten, Emanuel. 'Mejlen som avslöjar Gieseckes inflytande', *Expressen*, 11 August 2020, <https://www.expressen.se/nyheter/qs/mejlen-som-avslojar-gieseckes-inflytande-over-coronaplanen1/> accessed 15 August 2020.

8 Farmbrough, Heather. 'Why Sweden's approach to coronavirus may not be what you think', *Forbes*, 14 May 2020, <https://www.forbes.com/sites/heatherfarmbrough/2020/05/14/why-swedens-approach-to-coronavirus-may-not-be-what-you-think/#159> accessed 2 June 2020.

9 Ray, John. 'Is Sweden's decision not to have a coronavirus lockdown a fatal mistake?' ITV News, 29 April 2020, <https://www.itv.com/news/2020-04-29/is-sweden-s-lack-of-coronavirus-lockdown-a -fatal-mistake/> accessed 2 June 2020.

10 Nelson, Fraser. 'Sweden tames its R number without lockdown', *The Spectator*, 4 May 2020, <https://www.spectator.co.uk/article/sweden-tames-its-r-number-without-lockdown> accessed 11 June 2020.

11 Farmbrough, as note 8

12 Interview, *Andrew Marr Show*, BBC, Sunday 26 April 2020, <https://www.bbc.co.uk/programmes/p08bjwp0> accessed 5 June 2020. At the time, Andrew Marr had been a popular news and current affairs broadcaster with BBC.

13 Farmbrough, as note 8.

14 Marr interview, as note 12, and, 'Löfven: Sverige har haft för dålig beredskap', *Svenska Dagbladet*, 9 April 2020, <https://www.svd.se/stefan-lofven-vi-har-inte-lyckats-skydda-vara-aldre> accessed 1 February 2022.

15 Ibid.

16 Ibid.

17 'Public agencies and how they are governed. Ministerial rule prohibited in Sweden', How Sweden is governed. Government Offices of Sweden, Stockholm, 2 March 2015, <https://government.se/how-sweden-is-governed/public-agencies-and-how-they-are-goverened/> accessed 6 June 2020.

18 Marr interview, as note 12.

19 Ray, as note 9.

20 Cuthbertson, Anthony. 'Coronavirus tracked: Charting Sweden's disastrous no- lockdown strategy', *Independent*, 1 June 2020, using data from Our World in Data, COVID-19 dataset, Global Change Data Lab, <https://www.independent.co.uk/news/world/europe/coronavirus-lockdown-sweden-death-rate-worst-country-covid-19-a9539206.html> accessed 14 December 2021.

21 Ibid.

Sweden's COVID-19 Mortality and R-Rate

Statistics, March 2020

Critics of Sweden's seemingly unique approach had the statistics to back them up. On 25 March 2020, Sweden had recorded the highest number of deaths per million per day in the world (in a rolling seven-day average), with 1.59 victims. Iran had recorded 1.58, and the UK 1.23.

A few days later, on 30 March, Sweden with 3.53 deaths per million per day (in a rolling seven-day average) would be overtaken by the UK with 3.54. Throughout April, the UK would widen the gap between them until Peru took the unenviable first place on 1 May with 9.72, with the UK at 9.6, and Sweden with 7.04. It went without saying of course that among all the Nordic countries, Sweden had the highest number of deaths, and with a large margin. On 31 March, Sweden had recorded 3.96 deaths per million per day (in a rolling seven-day average), while Denmark had recorded 1.43 deaths on that measure, Norway 0.71, and Finland 0.41. Iceland had recorded none.[1]

On the measure of cumulative confirmed COVID-19 deaths per million people, Sweden had again been out in front on 31 March with 37.89, the highest in the world, with the UK second highest with 36.02. Denmark had recorded 15.48 cumulative deaths per million, Iceland 5.83, Norway 7.14, and Finland 3.06.[2]

Actual deaths from COVID-19 in each of these countries – since 31 December 2019 – were, Sweden 385 from a population of 10 million, Denmark 90 from a population of 5.75 million, Norway 39 from a population of 5.4 million, and Finland 17 from a population of 5.5 million. In Iceland 2 people had died from of a population of 0.34 million.[3]

Statistics, April–June 2020

At the end of April 2020, Sweden's numbers remained strikingly higher than those of its neighbours.

The number of deaths per million per day in Sweden (in a rolling seven-day average) was 7.94, in Denmark it was 1.43, in Finland it was 1, and in Norway 0.42. In Iceland, there had been none. In Sweden, cumulative confirmed COVID-19 deaths per million people at the end of April numbered 254.52, while in Denmark it was 77.75, Norway 38.42, and Finland 38.03.[4]

In May, Sweden had one of the highest COVID-19 death rates in Europe with 7.3 deaths per million per day (13 May) in a rolling seven-day average and had earlier overtaken the UK which recorded 6.65 deaths per million per day (10 May). Well into May and early-June, central and south American countries were registering some of the highest death rates in the world. Peru would record 17.26 daily new deaths per million in a rolling seven-day average (5 June), Brazil 4.77, Mexico 4.12. On that day, Sweden recorded 4.06. In Europe on 5 June, 0.39 deaths per million per day had been recorded, and in the EU 0.18.[5]

As far as the cumulative death toll was concerned, on 5 June Sweden had recorded 4,639 deaths, the USA 112,321 (more than one quarter of the world total 416,001), the UK 38,505, and Italy 33,774. In Europe as a whole, 175,958 had died, and in the EU 127,812. On 5 June, Sweden's cumulative death toll (4,639) had overtaken that recorded by China (4,634).[6]

One of the reasons for Sweden's high death toll in comparison to the rest of Scandinavia was the extent to which the disease had spread to care homes, particularly in Stockholm – a point referred to by Isabella Lövin in her conversation with Andrew Marr. When asked if there was not some fear in Sweden that the country's approach might have been just too relaxed, especially when comparing its death rate with that in neighbouring countries, Lövin replied by referring to the strategy of protecting the elderly and the most vulnerable and admitting that Sweden was faced with 'a great problem in care homes'.[7]

Social and Cultural Differences Affecting the Swedish Death Rate

In Sweden, COVID-19 had spread faster in multigenerational households (households including both those older than seventy and those under fifteen). Additionally, locations with higher shares of immigrants had been more vulnerable to the virus.[8]

These locations were characterised by greater overcrowding and higher rates of multigenerational households, lower incomes, people working in frontline occupations, or who lacked language skills to understand the information given out by health authorities. In early-March 2020, there were suggestions that the Somali community had been hit hard due to a lack of public health information available in Somali.[9]

In its weekly report – taken from data over 6–12 April 2020 – the public health agency had noted that some population groups had been infected with and died from COVID-19 in greater numbers than other groups. After cross-matching personal data in laboratory-confirmed cases with personal data held by Statistics Sweden (*Statistikmyndigheten, SCB*), analysis showed that several countries of birth were over-represented among those infected or dying when compared with their representation in the population overall.[10]

The largest over-representation was indeed among those born in Somalia, accounting for 4.8 per cent of morbidity and mortality, but from a community representing less than 1 per cent of the population (0.84 per cent). Indeed, of the first ten deaths in Stockholm, six occurred among the Somali community.[11]

The report from the public health agency had come just after a survey by Stockholm health authorities which showed that the virus was hitting immigrant communities in the city's suburbs the hardest. The figures revealed that up to 6 April the Rinkeby-Kista borough area had 238 known cases of the virus and that Spånga-Tensta had 144. These figures equalled 47 cases per 10,000 and 37 cases per 10,000 inhabitants respectively, numbers which were well above the then average of 13 infections for every 10,000.[12]

Some of Stockholm's suburbs were immigrant-dense with up to 80 per cent of residents having been foreign-born, indeed more than half of the city's Somalis lived in just one district – Rinkeby, often referred to as 'Little Mogadishu'. Crowding and interacting multigenerational households were quite common, as were low incomes, and the potential for exposure to the virus was high. At the same time, it had been difficult to put in place social measures and initiatives – such as offering accommodation for elderly people to help them self-isolate – because of the fear of stigmatizing immigrant communities.[13]

Many of the staff in Stockholm's care homes and nursing homes, or who were home carers visiting the elderly in their own homes, had travelled in public transport from some of the worst affected suburbs and had been more likely to be living with older generations of their families. Also, many staff were on insecure contracts, often working in several care homes at once, and finding it more difficult to stay at home if they developed symptoms.[14] With the sheltering of the elderly and the vulnerable being one of the objectives of policy, the significant death rate in the care home sector was one area in which Tegnell was prepared to admit failures.[15]

Outside Stockholm and second city Gothenburg, population density for its 10.23 million people was low. Sweden had space and was the third largest country in Europe. More Swedes lived alone – formed single person households – than in any other country, and many preferred to keep a physical and social distance from other people.[16] According to Eurostat figures (2016), more than half of Swedish households were made up of only one person (52 per cent of all households). Compared to the EU average of 26, the most common age to move out from of the parental home in Sweden was 18 and 19.[17]

Swedes had given each other wide physical space long before the coronavirus pandemic hit the country.[18] Indeed, the former prime minister and former foreign minister Carl Bildt had himself joked that 'Swedes, especially of the older generation, have a genetic disposition to social distancing'.[19]

Culturally in Sweden, different generations had not interacted as much as they had done, traditionally, in Italy and so this meant less of a risk of younger people passing on the virus to the elderly in a household. While the interaction of different generations could not really have relevance in any comparison between Italian and Swedish death rates (the former so low, the latter so high), it did have relevance in explaining why a disproportionate number of Sweden's COVID-19 deaths occurred within the country's Somali community, whose members tended to live in cramped accommodation in poorer neighbourhoods, with more multigenerational mingling and interacting and less access to government information.[20]

When asked by Marr if the country's lower population density, high proportion of single person households, and its own cultural factors had made a difference to the Swedish approach and acceptance of it, Lövin said that, when compared with other countries, these factors along with the level of wealth and welfare that people enjoyed in Sweden made it easier for the population to follow the advice of authorities and to distance or isolate themselves. Swedes were privileged in being able to do this without hardship; something totally impossible to do in developing countries where multigenerational families were the norm, and where life was lived in proximity to others, and in poverty.[21]

Sweden's R-Rate

Sweden had been described as the world's COVID-19 'outrider' and COVID-19 'outlier'. It had earned these appellatives by pursuing social distancing but rejecting mandatory lockdown, and by keeping part of its school system open, along with its bars and restaurants.[22]

While the Swedish death toll was well above that of neighbouring Denmark, Norway, and Finland, hospitals had not been pushed to breaking point. Indeed, there had been 20–30 per cent spare capacity in intensive care beds after efforts early in the crisis to double the number of beds,[23] and by early-June a field hospital set up by Region Stockholm in Älvsjö, aided by the armed forces and national agencies, was set to be dismantled without having received a single patient. Well into May, the number of patients in critical condition had been falling and Sweden's R-number, or reproduction number, had dropped to below 1.

The R-number was a measurable value that was used by countries to judge the success, or otherwise, of lockdown. An R-number of 1 meant that an infected person would pass the virus to one other person, an R-number of 2 meant two others would be infected, an R-number of 3 meant the infection of three others, and so on upwards. The objective was to push R below 1, and the strong international interest in seemingly maverick Sweden was to determine whether or not voluntary lockdowns worked just as well as enforced ones, and if they could keep the virus at a manageable level with lower social and economic cost.[24]

According to modelling conducted by Imperial College, London, shielding, voluntary social distancing, and even school closures, made little difference to the R-number and spread of the virus. It was lockdown that made the game-changing difference. Modelling for the UK with measures such as self-isolation for those with symptoms and social distancing encouraged for everyone, showed that during early- to mid-March the infection rate or R-number would hover just below 4. In other words, every person infected with COVID-19 would give it to 3–4 others. With the introduction of lockdown measures in the Imperial College model, the R-number would show a sharp drop to 1 and below 1 by end-March and into early-April.[25]

As described in the Imperial College multi-authored *Report 13: Estimating the number of infections and the impact of non-pharmaceutical interventions on COVID-19 in 11 European countries* (30 March) the modelling for Sweden based on assumptions for the UK had been dire. The report warned that a rejection of lockdown was likely to leave the virus rampant with an R-number possibly as high as 3 or 4. The findings were interpreted by academics and scientists in Lund and Uppsala as meaning a caseload for the healthcare system of up to 370,000 COVID-19 patients, with 40,000 deaths by 1 May and almost 100,000 by June.[26] As it turned out, the modelling was wrong. By 5 June, and as shown earlier, Sweden had recorded 4,639 deaths. On the date of publication of the Imperial College report, 30 March, Sweden had 4,359 confirmed cases,[27] a long way from the caseload of 370,000 patients predicted by the English model.

By early-May, the R-number in the UK had been estimated at 0.8 (plus or minus 0.2 points), described as an achievement of lockdown. By comparison, the Swedish R-number had dropped to 0.85 (plus or minus a smaller 0.02 points), an achievement surely of voluntary lockdown.

Chapter 4 will describe the gradual easing of the measures and will look at testing and contact-tracing, and statistics and spikes during the summer months. Differences in mortality between Sweden and its neighbours had implications for new travel agreements. What were these? Why had the WHO designated Sweden a 'hotspot' and high-risk country? On spikes and the spread of infection, was Sweden going against the European trend a showing a decline in spread?

Notes

1 'Daily new confirmed COVID-19 deaths per million people, March 31, 2020', also for 30 March, and 1 May, using Johns Hopkins University CSSE as a source, Our World in Data, COVID-19 dataset, <https://ourworldindata.org> accessed 14 December 2021. International comparative coronavirus statistics presented in this and other chapters had been taken between 14–20 December 2021 from data compiled by Johns Hopkins University (JHU) / Centre for Systems Science and Engineering, CSSE, from January 2020 onwards and as presented on the OWID website 'Our World in Data' (Oxford Martin School / University of Oxford / Global Change Data Lab). As with the upkeep of any large international statistical dataset – offering unemployment figures, or GDP, or whatever—the JHU / CSSE was unlikely to have received relevant coronavirus statistics from national agencies, authorities, and governments simultaneously. Health agencies and governments around the world published and reported their statistics on testing, confirmed cases, policy responses, hospitalizations, excess mortality, and vaccinations, at different times and in differing cycles, and researchers checking the OWID dataset regularly would have found changes in these – some slight, some significant – from one week to the next. Additionally, registration authorities might not have processed death certificates or other data for several days, or maybe weeks, creating lag in the data. These factors, and any number of other changes made to different national methods of recording over time, would have had an influence on the data published and might have accounted for any differences observed by researchers at different periods. It should be noted too that for several months in 2020, OWID had presented data compiled by the European Centre for Disease Control, ECDC, but from 30 November 2020, all data on confirmed cases and deaths and presented in OWID charts, maps, and tables were provided by JHU (References: 'Tracking Covid-19 excess deaths across countries', *The Economist*, 13 December 2021, and Ritchie Hannah. 'Our World in Data switches to Johns Hopkins University as our main data source for COVID-19 cases and deaths', 30 November 2020).

2 'Cumulative confirmed COVID-19 deaths per million people, March 31, 2020, Our World in Data, COVID-19 dataset, <https://ourworldindata.org> accessed 14 December 2021.

3 'Cumulative confirmed COVID-19 deaths, March 31, 2020, Our World in Data, COVID-19 dataset, <https://ourworldindata.org> and, 'Countries in the world by population (2020)', elaboration of UN data, Worldometer, <www.worldmeters.info> accessed 14 December 2021.

4 'Daily new confirmed COVID-19 deaths per million people, April 30, 2020', and, 'Cumulative confirmed COVID-19 deaths per million people, April 30, 2020', Our World in Data, COVID-19 dataset, <https://ourworldindata.org> accessed 14 December 2021.

5 'Daily new confirmed COVID-19 deaths per million people, May 10, May 13, and June 5, 2020', Our World in Data, COVID-19 dataset, <https://ourworldindata.org> accessed 15 December 2021.

6 'Cumulative confirmed COVID-19 deaths, June 5, 2020, Our World in Data, COVID-19 dataset, <https://ourworldindata.org> accessed 15 December 2021.

7 Interview, *Andrew Marr Show*, BBC, Sunday 26 April 2020, <https://www.bbc.co.uk/programmes/p08bjwp0> accessed 5 June 2020.

8 Florida, Richard. and Charlotta Mellander. 'The geography of Covid-19 in Sweden', p. 130, in *The annals of regional science*, Vol. 68, pp. 125–150, 2022, <https://doi.org/10.1007/s00168-021-01071-0> accessed 7 February 2025.

9 Ibid.

10 'Veckorapport on covid-19, vecka 15 (a report taken over 6–12 April 2020, week 15)', Folkhälsomyndigheten / Public Health Agency, 17 April 2020, <https://www.folkhalsomyndigheten.se/globalassets/statistik-uppfoljning/smittsamma-sjukdomar/veckorapporter-covid-19/2020/covid-19-veckorapport-vecka-15.pdf> accessed 1 July 2020.

11 Eaton, George. 'Trust is vital if you want to stop this disease', Anders Tegnell on leading Sweden's fight against Covid-19, p. 17 *New Statesman*, 23–29 October 2020, p. 16–17. Those born in Iraq, Syria, Finland, Türkiye, Iran, countries of the former-Yugoslavia, and Eritrea, were also over-represented ('Veckorapport on covid-19, vecka 15, as note 10).

12 Franssen, Anne Grietje. 'Why are there so many coronavirus cases in Stockholm's northern suburbs?' *The Local*, 9 April 2020, <https://thelocal.se/20200409/why-are-there-so-many-coronavirus-cases-in-stockholms-northern-suburbs> accessed 1 July 2020.

13 Rothschild, Natalie. 'The hidden flaws in Sweden's anti-lockdown strategy', *Foreign Policy*, 21 April 2020, <https://foreignpolicy.com/2020/04/21/sweden-coronavirus-anti-lockdown-immigrants/> accessed 3 July 2020, and Gorokov, S. A. *et al*. 'Little Mogadishu in Stockholm, or Apartheid with a friendly face in Sweden', pp. 57–65, *Asia & Africa today*, No. 3, 2024, Russian Centre for Science Information, <https://doi.org/10.31857/S032150750030456-3> accessed 2 May 2025.

14 Farmbrough, Heather. 'Why Sweden's approach to coronavirus may not be what you think', *Forbes*, 14 May 2020, <https://www.forbes.com/sites/heatherfarmbrough/2020/05/14/why-swedens-approach-to-coronavirus-may-not-be-what-you-think/#159> accessed 2 June 2020.

15 Ray, John. 'Is Sweden's decision not to have a coronavirus lockdown a fatal mistake?' ITV News, 29 April 2020, <https://www.itv.com/news/2020-04-29/is-sweden-s-lack-of-coronavirus-lockdown-a -fatal-mistake/> accessed 2 June 2020.

16 Farmbrough, as note 14.

17 'Over half of Sweden's households made up of one person', Eurostat, 5 September 2017, <https://ec.europa.eu/eurostat/web/products-eurostat-news/-/DDN-20170905-1?inheritRedirect=true> accessed 24 November 2020.

18 Savage, Maddy. 'Could the Swedish lifestyle help fight coronavirus?' Remote control, Covid-19, BBC, 28 March 2020, <http://www.bbc.com/worklife/article/20200328-how-to-self-isolate-what-we-can-learn-from-sweden> accessed 24 November 2020.

19 'Why Swedes are not yet locked down', *The Economist*, 4 April 2020, <https://economist.com/europe/2020/04/04/why-swedes-are-not-yet-locked-down> accessed 23 October 2020.

20 Pancevski, Bojan. and Dominic Chopping. 'Inside Sweden's radically different approach to the coronavirus', *The Wall Street Journal*, 30 March 2020. <https://www.wsj.com/articles/inside-swedens-radically-different-approach-to-the-coronavirus-11585598175> accessed 26 April 2020.

21 Marr interview, as note 7.

22 Nelson, Fraser. 'Sweden tames its R number without lockdown', *The Spectator*, 4 May 2020, <https://www.spectator.co.uk/article/sweden-tames-its-r-number-without-lockdown> accessed 11 June 2020.

[23] Edwards, Catherine. 'As Europe comes out of lockdown, what lessons can be learned from Sweden?' *The Local*, 20 May 2020, <https://www.thelocal.se/20200520/as-europe-comes-out-of-lockdown-what-lessons-can-be-learned-from-sweden> accessed 12 June 2020.

[24] Nelson, as note 22.

[25] Ibid.

[26] Ibid.

[27] 'Cumulative confirmed COVID-19 cases, March 30, 2020', Our World in Data, COVID-19 dataset, <https://ourworldindata.org> accessed 15 December 2021.

Easing of Measures

Green Light to Domestic Travel – New Spike Around Gothenburg

Into June 2020, Sweden was moving to a new phase in its fight against the virus, and with thoughts perhaps turning to the Midsummer holidays and the traditional long Swedish shutdown, the government had given the green light to domestic travel again for those who were free from infection.

There had been good reasoning behind this step, not least the long-term sustainability of the Swedish approach which Tegnell had defended. People needed encouragement to get moving around the country again, and if the country were to retain a tourist industry as large as it had been before COVID-19, then the existing travel advice had to be changed. Hotels, campsites, and holiday villages had been hard hit, and the industry had been lobbying the government for relief. Arguing against the reasoning were the smaller devolved healthcare regions which were worried about how they would be able to cope with large numbers of sick tourists. Gotland – Sweden's holiday island in the Baltic – might have to be given extra support for healthcare.[1]

Meanwhile, just as the lifting of travel restrictions was being announced – taking effect from 13 June – Tegnell announced that there had been an unexpected spike in cases of the virus in Region Västra Götaland (a devolved council area composed of Gothenburg and the adjacent counties of Älvsborg, Bohuslän, and Skaraborg).[2] Several hospitals in the region had seen an increase in admissions, an obvious sign of greater community spread. In addition, there had been evidence from Telia – large Nordic-Baltic mobile network operator – that there had been a sharp rise in travelling. People were getting tired of working from home and keeping social distance. Nevertheless, when asked if it would be a good idea to keep travel restrictions in place for Region Västra Götaland and in parts of the very popular west coast – Bohuslän – the public health agency said that their preference was that the new travel advice apply to the country as a whole. The regional differences in cases were not so great that they created a risk for people moving from place to place. Neither regional spikes nor the continued spread of the infection was going to affect the new travel advice.[3]

Testing and Contact-Tracing

In another change in tack, and with yet another extra budget announcement after negotiations with coalition partners – the Centre Party and Liberals – Lena Hallengren, the minister for health and social affairs, said that an additional SEK 6 billion would be allocated to the regions to be used in a large testing and contact-tracing programme.

Hitherto, testing for COVID-19 had been slow, and a target of 100,000 tests a week set in April was still far from being reached. To avoid a second wave of infection, there would be a renewed focus on the testing and contact-tracing programme, and antibody tests, which would show who had had the virus before, were to be included in the programme.[4]

The testing programme would not be open to anyone who simply wanted a test but rather to everyone who showed COVID-19 symptoms, and who had undergone some form of medical examination first. Acting leader of the Centre Party, Anders W. Jonsson (leader Annie Lööf was on parental leave), argued that this was unnecessary and the wrong way to go. He was disappointed that administrative barriers were being put in the way of a quick start to testing and contact-tracing. Anyone with symptoms and who could have COVID-19 ought to be tested without any doctor or nurse being involved. Carrying out medical examinations would only add to the burden of the healthcare system.[5]

Hallengren had defended the slow implementation of mass testing and tracing, saying that the earlier focus had been on prioritizing the testing of those who were seriously ill, and the testing of healthcare personnel, but now the infection was in a phase which offered room for wider testing.[6]

Upper Secondary Schools and Universities Re-Open

Testing thus far had shown a low spread of infection among children and teenagers with fewer than 600 people aged under 20 years of age having tested positive for COVID-19. These findings offered some justification for the early decision to keep schools open for those under the age of sixteen (*grundskolor*).

Part of the reasoning behind schools remaining open for lower secondary and primary school-aged children was to ensure that key workers would be able to remain in post. Many parents however had been concerned about sending their children to school.[7]

Since the school-aged young were not believed to be major spreaders of COVID-19, nor a significant risk of developing serious illness if exposed to it, Johan Carlson, director-general at the public health agency, believed that there could no longer be any justification for the recommendation of distance learning for upper secondary schools (the over-16s) which had been in place since mid-March. So then, towards the end of May, Löfven and Carlson, and the education minister, Anna Ekström, announced that universities and upper secondary schools would reopen from 15 June. Since most students would leave again shortly after that for their summer holiday, the greater impact would be felt in the autumn term.[8]

Universities and other adult education institutions, and their students, were still expected to follow the other coronavirus restrictions and recommendations such as avoiding non-essential travel, the ban on public gatherings of more than fifty people and keeping in place social distance measures.[9]

Statistics, June–July 2020

As the government changed tack – on travel advice, testing, and the reopening of universities and upper secondary schools – its management of the emergency was being criticised more and more, and public confidence was starting to fall. The death toll had become much more serious.

While the virus had hit Sweden, Denmark, Finland, and Norway at roughly the same time, and although the countries were all – arguably – quite similar, outcomes had been different. Sweden's neighbours had all locked down quicker and to far greater degrees, hoping to gain some time by completely stopping the spread of infection. Sweden on the other hand had accepted a certain spread of infection, with the expectation that that the healthcare system would be able to cope. The result was that on the last day of June, Sweden had recorded 2.42 deaths per million per day (in a rolling seven-day average), Denmark and Norway each recorded 0.05, Finland 0.03, and Iceland 0. This compared with 0.86 in the UK and 1.58 in the USA. In Europe on 30 June, 0.49 deaths per million per day had been recorded, and in the EU 0.28. In South America, Peru had recorded 15.7, Chile 8.8, Mexico 4.82, and Brazil 4.64.[10]

As far as cumulative deaths were concerned, on 30 June Sweden had recorded 5,333 deaths, Denmark had recorded 605, Finland 328, Norway 250, and Iceland 10. In the UK, 40,479 deaths had been recorded, in the USA 127,365, in the EU 133,134, and in wider Europe 188,085.[11]

A month later, on 31 July, mortality rates had fallen markedly in Sweden 0.65 deaths per million per day (in a rolling seven-day average) were recorded compared to 0.21 in the UK and 3.32 in the USA. On this measure at the end of June, the Swedish rate had been between three and four times greater (at 2.42). In Europe continent-wide on 31 July, 0.4 deaths per million per day had been recorded, and in the EU 0.2. Peru had recorded 18.27, Brazil had gone up slightly to 4.83, Mexico had gone down to 4.43, while Chile had recorded 4.04 (almost half its rate end-June). In Denmark 0.05 deaths per million per day had been recorded, and in Norway, Finland, and Iceland, the figure was 0.[12]

The cumulative total of deaths recorded in Sweden on 31 July was 5,743, and in Denmark it was 615, in Finland 329, in Norway 255, and in Iceland still 10. In the UK, 41,274 deaths had been recorded, in the EU 136,136, in the USA 153,828, and in Europe as a whole 198,424.[13]

Nordic Green Light to Travel – Not to Sweden

The striking differences in mortality between Sweden and its Nordic neighbours in April and May would exclude Sweden from a new travel agreement reached between Denmark and Norway in May, coming as a blow to the Swedish government.

Sweden had pressed its neighbours not to exclude it from a border deal despite that higher rate of infection, but while Mette Frederiksen the Danish prime minister, recognized that Danes and Swedes had cross-border connections – family and other relationships, business and so on – their two countries were at different places in the fight against the virus and this had a bearing on border arrangements. Denmark was also opening its borders to tourists from Germany and Iceland. For the time being, Norway was only opening its borders to tourists from Denmark.[14]

The new agreement still held some restrictions. Travellers coming into Denmark from Norway, Germany and Iceland would have to show proof that they had a reservation at a hotel, holiday let, or campsite for a minimum of six nights somewhere other than in Copenhagen – no overnight staying in the capital – and they would be encouraged on a random basis to take a test for COVID-19. Norway would not be imposing any similar restrictions on Danish tourists. The new travel arrangements would come into effect on 15 June.[15]

Having reopened her country to Denmark, the Norwegian prime minister, Erna Solberg, said that talks had been underway with Sweden, Finland and Iceland about including them in the same 'travel bubble', and that the ultimate goal was a renewing of the common regulatory framework for the Nordic countries. The situation in Sweden had constituted the greatest hurdle, but a solution might be found for regions of the country that had a low level of infection. Travel restrictions against visitors from Sweden could be lifted on a regional basis provided that an adequate model could be found. Sweden and Finland could be included in the 'travel bubble' by 31 August.[16]

The E20 via the Öresund Bridge and through Sweden was one of the main road traffic routes from Copenhagen to Helsinki. Since 14 March 2020 and the imposition of stricter rules for entry into Denmark, the Öresund Bridge had been partially closed, twenty years since its formal opening to traffic. While the bridge remained open to freight traffic in both directions, and to private vehicular travel to Sweden, there were stricter rules for travel into Denmark from Sweden. Those wishing to travel to Denmark had to have a valid reason for doing so, such as living or working there, delivering vital goods, or holding Danish citizenship.[17] In April, the total traffic on the Öresund Bridge – motorcycles, cars, vans, and coaches – had been 190,827. This compared with 613,280 in April 2019. In May 2020 traffic had risen to 292,806, compared with 650,211 in the previous May.[18] A long six-kilometre queue of Danish traffic returning from Sweden after the weekend holiday marking Ascension Day (*Kristi himmelsfärdsdag*) in May had fuelled resentment in Sweden over Danes being able to travel freely into Sweden, while they were barred from travelling to Denmark without good reason.[19]

Just prior to the new rules between Denmark, Norway, Germany, and Iceland coming into effect, Finland announced that it too would be opening its borders on 15 June. The new Finnish arrangements applied not only to Denmark, Norway, and Iceland, but also Estonia, Latvia, and Lithuania. The concentration of COVID-19 in Sweden prevented it from being included.[20]

Green Light to Cross-Border Travel

Having already given the green light to domestic travel again in early-June, the Swedish foreign ministry announced that from 30 June guidance to avoid all non-essential travel to ten EU/EEA countries would be scrapped. The guidance – never a legally enforced ban – had been in place since mid-March and was extended in mid-May.

The countries to which travel had been given the green light were Belgium, Croatia, France, Greece, Iceland, Italy, Luxembourg, Portugal, Switzerland, and Spain. The list was not based on any assessment of COVID-19 risk in these countries, but on the fact that they had not introduced restrictions against Swedes. The other mainland Nordic countries (Denmark, Norway, and Finland) did not make it to the list because of the restrictions they had placed on travellers from Sweden. Advice against travel to other countries in the EU, the EEA, and the Schengen area – and that included Denmark, Norway, and Finland of course – would remain in place until at least 15 July.[21]

From 1 July, Brussels began a gradual lifting of restrictions on non-essential travel into the EU, easing restrictions at external borders for residents of several countries. These had been in place since 17 March, with extensions having been announced in April and in May. The criteria used to determine the countries for which the restrictions could be lifted covered: the epidemiological situation in the country, and whether it was above or below the EU average, and whether it showed a stable or decreasing trend in new cases; containment measures including physical distancing, testing and contact-tracing; and economic and social considerations. The list was to be reviewed and updated every two weeks.[22]

Based on the criteria and conditions set out, EU member states could start lifting travel restrictions at external borders for residents of: Algeria, Australia, Canada, Georgia, Japan, Montenegro, Morocco, New Zealand, Rwanda, Serbia, South Korea, Thailand, Tunisia, and Uruguay. China was to be on the list too, subject to confirmation of reciprocity.[23] Noticeable by its absence was the USA, but also excluded from the list were Brazil, India, and Russia. Until the end of the 'Brexit' transition period on 31 December 2020, UK nationals would be treated as EU citizens although, depending on which countries they might travel to in the EU, they could face having to go into quarantine when they got home again.

People from all the countries listed would be allowed to travel to Sweden for any purpose, including tourism. Although there were no quarantine rules in place for foreign visitors, and no requirement to prove negativity to coronavirus, travellers would be expected to follow Sweden's coronavirus health and safety guidelines.[24]

By mid-July, Denmark had become open to travel from regions of Sweden with low coronavirus infection rates – Region Blekinge, Region Kronoberg, and Region Skåne in the south, and Region Västerbotten in the north – and from regions bordering these if proof of a negative coronavirus test could be shown. Norway too had become open to travellers from Blekinge, Kronoberg, and Skåne, but was advising against non-essential travel to Sweden beyond these three regions, and for a quarantine of ten days on return if that occurred. Finland remained closed to non-essential travel from Sweden. Those returning from Sweden had to self-isolate for two weeks. All three countries permitted travel from Sweden if the purpose of the visit was to continue a serious relationship with someone, though self-isolation rules still applied.[25]

By mid-July too, guidance to avoid all non-essential travel to Germany, Poland and Andorra was lifted, with these three countries joining the ten already listed from 30 June, although guidance against travel to Switzerland was reintroduced temporarily. Other than those now twelve countries listed as open for travel, foreign ministry recommendations against non-essential journeys to countries in the EU, EEA, and Schengen area, as well as the UK and Switzerland, were extended until the end of July.[26]

In August, temporary bans were in place against people entering Sweden from Algeria, Montenegro, Morocco, and Serbia, other than for urgent family reasons, or for workers in key roles.

WHO – 'Hotspot' Sweden

After the pressure of having to explain the unexpected spike in cases in Västra Götaland, Tegnell and the whole Swedish approach to tackling coronavirus would come under yet more pressure during June, this time from the WHO. The new attack came just days before the scrapping of restrictions on non-essential travel to several EU/EEA countries and, to a degree, backed up the stance taken by Sweden's neighbours.

In a statement from the WHO Europe Office on 25 June – and as clarified by the Belgian physician and WHO regional director for Europe, Hans Kluge – Sweden had been classified as a COVID-19 high-risk country and placed on a list of eleven countries with accelerated transmissions that could overwhelm their health systems. Kluge had said that it was clear Sweden was still undergoing wide social spread of coronavirus.[27]

While the public health agency had achieved good results for which the WHO was appreciative of, the WHO considered the spread of COVID-19 as still problematic in Sweden, and Kluge urged the government and health authorities to continue to scale up measures to stop the spread of infection. Over the two weeks prior to the WHO statement, thirty countries had shown cumulative increases in new cases, and in eleven of them, including Sweden, the increases had been so noticeable that, if not taken care of, healthcare systems would be pushed to their limits. In the view of the WHO, Sweden was a high-risk country – a COVID-19 'hotspot'. The eleven hotspot countries were: Albania, Armenia, Azerbaijan, Bosnia and Herzegovina, Kazakhstan, Kosovo, Kyrgyzstan, Moldova, Northern Macedonia, Sweden, and Ukraine.[28]

In response, Tegnell said that the WHO assessment had been based on a misinterpretation of the statistics, and that the increase in new cases had been due to more people having been tested since a relaunch of the testing and contact-tracing programme earlier in the month. Into late-June, around 60,000 people had been tested compared to around 30,000 in May.[29] From all other measurable parameters, serious cases of COVID-19 were decreasing and the number of admissions to intensive care was low, and even deaths were starting to decline. Indeed, deaths occurring in Sweden at that point in late-June were no greater than in any normal year. He criticised the WHO for looking at only one set of statistics, and for not consulting with Sweden as to what might have lain behind the figures before making its assessment.[30]

A few days after the WHO statement, the UK had lifted blanket restrictions on non-essential travel overseas allowing Britons to travel to certain European countries without having to spend fourteen days in quarantine on their return. So-called 'travel corridors' or 'air bridges' would be put in place with a traffic light system classifying countries as green, amber, or red, depending on the prevalence of coronavirus in them. Sweden and Portugal were expected to be given a red light.[31]

New Spikes in Europe – July–August – New Green Light for Sweden

Well into the summer, in late-July, spikes in coronavirus infection in Europe particularly in Spain – in Aragon and Catalonia – but also showing in Belgium, France, Germany, Luxembourg, and Romania prompted the WHO to express fresh concerns. At the end of July, the continent of Europe had accounted for more than one in six of the 17.6 million cases across the world and remained the hardest hit in terms of deaths with 198,424 out of 711,989 globally since the emergence of COVID-19.[32]

Spain which had been hard-hit by coronavirus wanted to restart its economy and to encourage tourists to its beaches again, but France had issued a recommendation against travel to Catalonia – location of tourist hotspots such as Barcelona and the Costa Brava – and Norway had placed all of Spain on its 'red' list, along with Portugal, Andorra, Luxembourg, Bulgaria, Croatia, and Romania. The UK had also advised against non-essential travel to mainland Spain, and while exempting the Balearic Islands and the Canary Islands from that advice travellers would still have to self-isolate on their return. For many, travel to Spain now meant staying in isolation for between 10 and 14 days (depending on the home country of the traveller and its national advice).

While Norway had brought in new restrictions against travel to Spain, it had issued revised advice for travel from and to Sweden. Hitherto, only Region Blekinge, Region Kronoberg, and Region Skåne, had been exempted from travel restrictions, but from late-July Region Kalmar County, Region Östergötland, Region Örebro, and Region Värmland were exempted too. Travel to other parts of Sweden would still require self-isolation at home for ten days on return.[33]

This had been positive news for businesses in those parts of Värmland close to the Norwegian border – in small communities such as Charlottenberg and Töckfors – to which many Norwegians had traditionally come to shop instead of making the longer trip to Oslo. Värmland had readied itself for the expected onslaught of shopaholic Norwegians and could congratulate itself too for being the first border region to reopen. As soon as coronavirus had struck Sweden, the regional authorities had started tracking the infection, and now that the proportion of positive test results were lower than 5 per cent and there were fewer than 20 confirmed cases per 100,000 inhabitants over the last two weeks, there had been expectation that a relaxation in Norwegian restrictions would come.[34]

Earlier in the year, there had been a meeting of the Norwegian Institute of Public Health, NIPH (*Folkehelseinstituttet, FHI*) and Denmark's State Serum Institute (*Statens Serum Institut, SSI*) to discuss common criteria for Nordic travel. They had agreed that for travel to a Swedish region or county there had to be fewer than 20 cases per 100,000 inhabitants 'on average' over two weeks. Then, after agreement had been reached, Norway tightened its requirement to 20 cases per 100,000 inhabitants 'in total' (rather than on average) over the past two weeks. Subsequent collection of data led to differing results and a situation in which, in late-July, 'tighter' Norway had opened travel to 7 Swedish counties while Denmark had opened to 12.[35]

Sweden Against the Trend – Again

The spikes of infection in Europe had been described by Tegnell as 'worrying', particularly as it was happening in the summer rather than in the autumn as might have been expected. Globally the spread of infection continued to accelerate just as before.[36] Tegnell had argued throughout that the world faced a long and uncertain battle with the virus and that the only realistic way of coping in the long run – it was a marathon not a sprint – was to have kept society open and trained people to follow social and physical distancing. This had been the Swedish strategy.

About the situation in Sweden, Tegnell described this as being 'very positive' overall, and that the country was going against the European trend. The spread of infection continued to decline, with infection curves going down and the number of those seriously ill approaching zero.[37]

In spring, the public health agency had said that warmer summer weather could help to reduce the spread of infection, but in late-July Tegnell had, in part, re-evaluated that earlier assessment. The summer impact had not been as great as thought, and the decline in spread not as fast and quite late and did not appear to be linked to weather. Autumn presented some concerns, he said.[38]

Tegnell had earlier added to the debate on the matter of immunity to COVID-19 and how long that lasted. People who had recovered from the coronavirus were likely to be immune for six months, whether they had antibodies or not. So far, no cases of people falling ill twice from COVID-19 had been reported, he said, hence the assessment that 'if you do get COVID-19 you are immune, even if you don't develop antibodies'.[39]

In new guidance, the public health agency said that, though social distancing rules must still apply, it was safe for individuals who had been infected to come into contact with people in high-risk groups.[40]

Tegnell had also presented several different scenarios for the future trajectory of the pandemic in Sweden. The most likely was that the country would see around 3,000 more deaths related to the virus, but a worst-case scenario could see a further 5,800 deaths. A likely scenario was that Sweden would experience clusters of new cases which would then quickly subside.[41]

At the end of July, Tegnell and Hallengren advised that everyone who was able to work from home should continue to do so throughout the autumn, a continuation of the guideline that had been in place since mid-March. This would help to reduce congestion on the public transport networks, particularly for service workers and medical staff who could not work from home. Tegnell had been unable to say when employees could expect to return to work, though it was likely to be a gradual process. He had added that it was 'an interesting question' as to whether the country would ever be able to go back to working 'in exactly the same way as before'.[42]

In addition to the advice to continue working from home – if able to – other official recommendations remained as before: stay at home if at all sick (even a mild cough or sore throat), keep social distance, practice good hygiene, and avoid non-essential visits to the elderly or to hospitals.

Although the public health agency had not recommended the wearing of masks by the public – even though much of the rest of Europe had done so – and had cited the lack of conclusive scientific proof of its efficacy, the Karolinska Institute was going to recommend mask-wearing in certain situations when medical teaching staff and students returned to campus for the autumn semester. The decision was likely to spark renewed debate within Sweden's medical science community and across the country at large. On the one hand Tegnell had said that a review of guidelines on mask-wearing was not being considered – against the trend again – and on the other the Sweden-based ECDC (the EU agency with headquarters in Solna, Stockholm) and the Geneva-based WHO had said that there were situations where mask-wearing might be a good addition to other measures. Mask-wearing might be effective when a local spike was recorded, where crowding couldn't be avoided, and where the epidemiology was moving in an unfavourable direction – Tegnell had also said.[43]

After a slow and steady decline in new daily deaths since a peak in mid-April, the public health agency had been able to announce on 7 August that no new coronavirus deaths had been reported for the first time since March.[44] While elsewhere a resurgence of coronavirus cases was being battled with, cases had actually dropped sharply in Sweden over the summer with a slight rise just prior to schools reopening again after the summer holidays. The return to school had inevitably brought more crowded public transport, though online lessons, staggered start times, and changes to bus schedules had helped mitigate this.[45]

According to the agency, the R-number – one of the key indicators of the coronavirus infection rate – remained at a safe level in Sweden, despite an increase in cases in some cities and regions as students had returned to school, college, and university. On 24 September, the Swedish R-number had been estimated at 0.89. It had peaked in March at an estimated 1.69 and had been falling since then to stabilize at around 1.0 between early-April and mid-June. On 15 September it had reached 1.15, and back to 1.0 on 20 September before dropping below 1 on 24 September.[46] Across all four nations of the UK around the same time, the R-number ranged between 1.3 and 1.6.[47]

Chapter 5 will focus on a second wave of the virus driving across Europe, new lockdowns, and regional differences. There will also be focus on the second wave in Sweden and new restrictions, autumn statistics, vaccines, and a new variant of COVID-19. Had Sweden been right all along, enabling citizens to mitigate the risks minimizing the need for government-led interventions? What measures did Sweden put in place to counter the new wave? What had other EU member states put in place to stem the new rise in cases? As the second wave of coronavirus swept across Europe, and as all of Sweden's regions introduced stricter restrictions based on public health agency recommendations, wasn't it the case that there was more that united the approaches taken by the different Scandinavian countries than which divided them? And what was the controversy around Danish and Swedish mink farms?

Notes

1 Stenberg, Ewa. 'Löfven pressas allt mer i coronakrisen', *Dagens Nyheter*, 4 June 2020, <https://www.dn.se/nyheter/sverige//ewa-stenberg-lofven-pressas-allt-mer-i-coronakrisen/> accessed 8 June 2020.

2 There had been a two-decade long process of regional reform in Sweden. It had begun with an experimental reform in 1999 when two county councils in the south were merged to form the new Region Skåne with Malmö as its main centre. In the west, three county councils formed Region Västra Götaland with Gothenburg as its main centre. In addition to an increase in size of the regional authority, the experimental reform also included devolution to the of the responsibility for physical planning, culture, environment, infrastructure and other regional development issues. In 2010, the reform became permanent and from 1 January 2019, all country councils, including Gotland, became regions (Gotland becoming Gotland Municipality). The Sami parliament (Sámidiggi, or Sametinget) is a special regional governing unit inaugurated in 1993, and the Sami people had been recognized by the *Riksdag* as a separate people in 1977, and by the Constitution in 2011.

3 Herold, Lovis. 'Kraftig ökning av antalet covid-19-fall i Västra Götalandsregionen', *Dagens Nyheter*, 4 June 2020, <https://www.dn.se/nyheter/sverige/kraftig-okning-av-antalet-covid-19-fall-i-vastra-gotalandsregionen/> accessed 8 June 2020.

4 Rosén, Hans. 'Alla med symptom ska testas – regeringen satsar 6 miljarder', *Dagens Nyheter*, 4 June 2020, <https://www.dn.se/nyheter/sverige/alla-med-symtom-ska-testas-regeringen-satsar-6-miljarder/> accessed 8 June 2020.

[5] Ibid.

[6] Ibid.

[7] 'Sweden to reopen universities and schools for over-16s', *The Local*, 29 May 2020, <https://www.thelocal.se/20200529/is-sweden-about-to-reopen-its-universities-and-schools-for-over-16s> accessed 10 June 2020.

[8] Ibid.

[9] Ibid.

[10] 'Daily new confirmed COVID-19 deaths per million people, June 30, 2020, Our World in Data, COVID-19 dataset, <https://ourworldindata.org> accessed 15 December 2021.

[11] 'Cumulative confirmed COVID-19 deaths, June 30, 2020, Our World in Data, COVID- 19 dataset, <https://ourworldindata.org> accessed 15 December 2021.

[12] Daily new confirmed COVID-19 deaths per million people, July 31, 2020, Our World in Data, COVID-19 dataset, <https://ourworldindata.org> accessed 15 December 2021.

[13] 'Cumulative confirmed COVID-19 deaths, July 31, 2020, Our World in Data, COVID- 19 dataset, <https://ourworldindata.org> accessed 15 December 2021.

[14] 'Denmark and Norway strike tourist border deal…without Sweden', *The Local*, 29 May 2020, <https://www.thelocal.se/20200529/denmark-and-norway-open-borders-for-eachothers-tourists> accessed 10 June 2020.

[15] Ibid.

[16] Ibid.

[17] 'Information regarding coronavirus', Øresundsbron, <https://www.oresundsbron.com/en/info/information-vedrorende-coronavirus> accessed 10 June 2020.

[18] The figures are taken from the traffic statistics of Øresundsbron, <https://www.oresundsbron.com/en/traffic-stats> accessed 22 June 2020.

[19] *The Local*, 29 May 2020, as note 14.

[20] 'Finland to open border to Norway and Denmark…but not to Sweden', *The Local*, 11 June 2020, <https://www.thelocal.se/20200611/finland-to-open-border-to-norway-and-denmarkbut-not-sweden> accessed 14 June 2020.

[21] 'Sweden gives green light to travel to ten countries from July', *The Local*, 17 June 2020, <https://www.thelocal.se/20200617/sweden-updates-international-travel-guidance-heres-what-it-means-for-you> and, Press release, Ministry for Foreign Affairs, 17 June 2020, <https://government.se/press-releases/2020/06/the-mfa-has-extended-the-advice-against-travel/> accessed 29 June 2020.

[22] 'Council agrees to start lifting travel restrictions for residents of some third countries', Press release, European Council / Council of the European Union, 30 June 2020, <https://www.consilium.europa.eu/en/press/press-releases/2020/06/30/council-agrees-to-start-lifting-travel-restrictions-for-residents-of-some-third-countries/> accessed 1 July 2020.

[23] Ibid.

[24] Löfgren, Emma. 'Sweden announces new exceptions to non-EU travel ban', *The Local*, 2 July 2020, <https://www.thelocal.se/20200702/sweden-expected-to-reveal-next-steps-for-non-eu-entry-ban> accessed 3 July 2020.

[25] 'Long distance relationships: What are the rules for travel to and from Sweden?', *The Local*, 14 July 2020, <https://www.thelocal.se/20200714/long-distance-relationships-what-are-the-rules-for-coming-to-sweden> accessed 17 July 2020.

[26] 'Sweden lifts travel warning for another three countries', *The Local*, 15 July 2020, <https://www.thelocal.se/20200715/sweden-lifts-recommendations-against-travel-to-another-three-countries> accessed 17 July 2020.

[27] Lagerwall, Katerina. and Dahl, Amanda. 'WHO backar delvis om Sverige som högriskland', *Dagens Nyheter*, 26 June 2020, <https://www.dn.se/nyheter/sverige/anders-tegnell-whos-varning-for-sverige-totalt-felaktig/> accessed 28 June 2020.

28 Ibid.

29 Bjarnefors, Stefan. and Dahl, Amanda. 'WHO: Smittspridningen stabil i Sverige', *Dagens Nyheter*, 26 June 2020, <https://www.dn.se/nyheter/sverige/who-backar-om-coronakritik/> accessed 28 June 2020.

30 Lagerwall, as note 27.

31 'Coronavirus: UK to open up European holidays from 6 July', *BBC News*, 27 June 2020, <https://www.bbc.co.uk/news/business-53199089> accessed 29 June 2020.

32 'Cumulative confirmed COVID-19 deaths, July 31, 2020', Our World in Data, COVID- 19 dataset, <https://ourworldindata.org> accessed 15 December 2021.

33 Karp, Ossi. 'Norge ger klartecken för ytterligare fyra Svenska regioner', *Dagens Nyheter*, 24 July 2020, <https://www.dn.se/nyheter/sverige/norge-kan-ge-klartecken-for-flera-svenska-regioner/> accessed 28 July 2020.

34 Ibid.

35 'Why is Norway tougher than Denmark on travel to Sweden?' *The Local*, 27 July 2020, <https://www.thelocal.se/20200727/why-are-norways-rules-for-travel-to-sweden-stricter-than-denmarks> accessed 28 July 2020.

36 Olsson, Gustav. and Amanda Dahl. 'Sverige går emot ökande smittotrend i Europa', *Dagens Nyheter*, 28 July 2020, <https://www.dn.se/nyheter/sverige/sverige-gar-emot-okande-smittotrend-i-europa/> accessed 29 July 2020.

37 Ibid.

38 Ibid.

39 'Immunity to Covid-19 lasts six months, says the man leading Sweden's fight against the disease', *The Telegraph*, 21 July 2020, <https://www.telegraph.co.uk/global-health/science-and-disease/immunity-covid-19-lasts-six-months-says-man-leading-swedens/> accessed 29 July 2020.

40 Ibid.

41 Ibid.

42 'Sweden urges employees to keep working from home throughout the autumn', *The Local*, 30 July 2020, <https://www.thelocal.se/20200730/Sweden-announces-new-guidelines-public-transport-work-home> accessed 3 August 2020.

43 'Swedish university tells staff and students to wear masks if distancing can't be maintained', *The Local*, 13 August 2020, <https://www.thelocal.se/20200813/swedish-university-the-effectiveness-of-face-masks-can-no-longer-be-disputed> accessed 15 August 2020.

44 'Why Sweden's total coronavirus death toll decreased on Friday', *The Local*, 7 August 2020, <https://www.thelocal.se/20200807/no-new-coronavirus-deaths-reported-in-sweden> accessed 10 August 2020.

45 'Swedish public transport operators brace for end of summer holidays', *The Local*, 12 August 2020, <https://www.thelocal.se/20200812/swedish-public-transport-operators-brace-for-end-of-summer-holidays> and, 'How Sweden's upper secondary schools are adapting to coronavirus', *The Local*, 11 August 2020, <https://www.thelocal.se/20200811/how-are-swedens-upper-secondary-schools-adapting-to-coronavirus> accessed 3 October 2020.

46 'What do we know about Sweden's R-number as coronavirus cases rise?' *The Local*, 1 October 2020, using data from the Swedish Public Health Agency, <https://thelocal.se/what-do-we-know-about-Swedens-r-number-as-coronavirus-cases-rise> accessed 4 October 2020.

47 'Covid-19 in the UK: How many coronavirus cases are there in your area?' *BBC News*, 5 October 2020, <https://www.bbc.co.uk/news/uk-51768274> accessed 5 October 2020.

New Normal

'Once-in-a-Century' Health Crisis

As spikes continued to be recorded across Europe into August 2020, the talk was of a second wave of coronavirus – as if the first had ever gone away.

Many countries that believed they were past the worst were now grappling with new outbreaks. In a statement from Geneva the WHO said that the pandemic was 'a once-in-a-century health crisis' and the effects from it would 'be felt for decades to come'. The WHO warned of the risk of 'response fatigue' as the disease placed continued social and economic pressure on countries.[1]

In France where the virus had been 'circulating more actively, with an increased loss of distancing and barrier measures', there was a risk of the country losing control. In Germany, the Marburger Bund – the largest professional association of doctors in the country and in Europe – claimed that Germany was already contending with a second wave of COVID-19 and risked squandering its early successes. In Denmark where the number of infections was rising and where a new phase in easing of lockdown was due to be discussed in parliament and by the government, Kåre Mølbak, the state epidemiologist at SSI, said he could not recommend proceeding to the next phase.[2] In the UK, local spikes had arisen in Leicester, the Blackburn area, Bradford, Oldham, Peterborough, Preston, Rochdale, and other areas in England, and in the city of Aberdeen, Scotland. Into September, Glasgow and two surrounding districts faced a local lockdown.

On the other side of the world, in Australia, where lockdown restrictions had been easing since May, the state of Victoria had re-imposed tight restrictions, and border closures were put in place between neighbouring states after a spiralling outbreak of the disease in Melbourne, caused by a breakdown in the isolation programme for returning travellers. In New Zealand, which had seen near elimination of the virus by end-May, and which had passed one hundred and two days without a locally transmitted case, a sudden local spike in Auckland, the largest city, brought new lockdown. In Vietnam, where no new infections had been recorded for three months, the country's first death occurred end-July, and an outbreak began in Da Nang a week before. In Hong Kong, a rise in cases had been cited as the reason for postponement of parliamentary elections scheduled for September, and a tightening of restrictions. India had also experienced a rise in new cases, and more than 2 million had been recorded in the country since the pandemic broke out. The virus had been spreading from the vast cities of Delhi and Mumbai to the more underdeveloped rural areas where fragile health systems were not coping.

Statistics, August–September 2020

Six months after the WHO had declared coronavirus to be public health emergency (a PHEIC), and when there had been fewer than 100 cases and no deaths outside China, by the beginning of August there were 17.86 million cases and 718,142 deaths across the world.[3]

On the measure of daily new confirmed cases per million people (on a rolling seven-day average) at the start of August, the USA and countries in Central America and the Caribbean were suffering worst with Panama recording 245.15 cases on that measure, Brazil 209.19, the USA 188.79, Colombia 182.2, Dominican Republic 137.19, Peru 135.03, and so on. Russia had recorded 37.75, India 37.43, and Iran 30.1.[4]

In Europe on the measure of daily new cases per million (on a rolling seven-day average), Luxembourg had recorded 135.92, Kosovo 131.22, Bosnia and Herzegovina 92.32, Serbia 62.99, Romania 62.98, Andorra 51.71, Spain 49.21, and Belgium 45.13, followed by Malta, Russia, Bulgaria, and then Sweden at 21.93, and a spike in Iceland caused 20.8 cases in that metric.[5]

There were no deaths from COVID-19 recorded in Sweden on 1 August, though there were four on 4 August. Throughout much of July, Denmark, Norway, Finland, and Iceland had recorded none, or perhaps one.

On 31 August, the cumulative total of deaths recorded in Sweden was 5,821, and in Denmark it was 624, in Finland 336, in Norway 264, and Iceland still 10. In the UK, after a revision of counting strategy in mid-August which knocked thousands from figures published earlier, 41,589 deaths had been recorded, in the USA 183,383, in the EU 140,056, and in Europe as a whole, 208,110.[6]

There had been no deaths from COVID-19 recorded in Sweden on 31 August, and none in Denmark, Norway, Iceland, or Finland.

As August came to a close and as autumn beckoned, some European countries continued to register growth in COVID-19 cases, and governments responded with a tightening of restrictions and safety measures. France and Italy had recorded large jumps, and the French prime minister, Jean Castex, said that the country was experiencing an 'undeniable surge' and that the epidemic 'could become exponential'. Indeed, the R-rate in France was now at 1.4, and cases were rising as fast as they had done in the early stage of the pandemic. Meanwhile in Spain, Germany and the UK, daily numbers were relatively stable, though the German government rejected calls for a relaxation in restrictions. As schools began to open across Europe for the autumn term, Hans Kluge at the WHO said that Europe was entering a 'tricky moment', at the same time stressing that schools were not a 'main contributor' to the spread.[7] In the last week of August, Spain became the first European country to record more than 450,000 cases of COVID-19 (though Russia spanning Europe and Asia had recorded over 990,000 cases).[8]

Well into the autumn month of September, and as new coronavirus cases had doubled over two weeks in more than half of the EU member states, Kluge said that the surging figures should serve as a wake-up call. A very serious situation was unfolding as weekly cases exceeded those reported during the first peak in March. Because the largest proportion of newly recorded cases was among younger people less likely to be severely impacted by the virus, hospital admissions and deaths had not yet seen a similar rise, but there were fears of many more cases of serious illness if the virus again spread to older and more vulnerable groups.[9]

According to Johns Hopkins University, by end-September almost 5 million confirmed cases and more than 222,000 fatalities had been recorded across Europe since the pandemic began. Across the world there had been almost 34 million confirmed cases and over 1 million deaths (that sober milestone having been passed 18–19 September 2020), with the USA, Brazil, India, Peru, Mexico, and the UK combined accounting for more than 610,000 of those deaths.[10]

On the measure of daily new cases per million (on a rolling seven-day average) at end-September a new range of countries were recording high rates of infection. Israel had recorded 632.69, Andorra 548.5, Bahrain 314.59, Montenegro 305.71, and Argentina 270.02, followed by Spain with 231.1. For comparison, Iceland had recorded 104.85, EU countries taken together had recorded 92.88, the UK 91.32, Denmark 89.47, and Hungary 89.13. Much lower down the table, Sweden had recorded 43.69 on the metric, Norway 19.6, and Finland 18.13.[11]

Since the start of the coronavirus outbreak, cumulative deaths across the Nordic countries by end-September were as follows: in Sweden 5,893, an increase of 72 since end-August; Denmark 650, an increase of 26; Finland 344, an increase of 8; Norway 274, an increase of 10; and Iceland 10, a static number since 19–20 April.[12]

Had Sweden Been Right All Along?

As autumn had embraced Europe, and as countries across the continent were gripped by a second wave of coronavirus infection, cities and regions again faced local lockdowns or other lesser restrictions – so called 'circuit breaker' lockdowns, or shorter periods of tighter rules and restrictions, or short sharp shocks.

From modelling performed in mid-March at the University of Edinburgh in Scotland (Mark Woolhouse, professor of infectious disease epidemiology), such a second lockdown in the UK had seemed inevitable. A team had modelled a lockdown ending in June which then showed a slow and 'initially imperceptible rise in cases over the summer, culminating in a second lockdown in September'. This scenario had been expected to play out because a lockdown was only a temporary fix, not a long-term solution. No matter how cautiously restrictions were relaxed, the epidemic was always likely to take off again.[13] As Tegnell had argued in Sweden in the spring, countries that had imposed tough and controlled lockdowns would have to end them sooner or later, facing the possibility of caseloads spiralling upwards again, out of control.

A doubling of cases every 7–14 days in mid-September was nothing like the doubling every 3–4 days experienced in mid-March however, and this slower rate had been anticipated. How populations were living now, six months into the pandemic, would prevent the virus from spreading as easily as it had before, and so the second wave of infection had been expected to be more like a second bump. Even so, a response of some kind was called for, something below the level of the harsh March lockdown.[14]

A targeted 'circuit breaker' driving down incidence over a short two-week period, say, would minimize disruption especially to healthcare provision and education, but also to businesses and services. Such a response had to focus on protecting the elderly and frail and had to be time-limited, come what may. The cure should not become worse than the disease.[15]

The longer-term strategy had to be a risk-based approach to living with COVID-19, and individuals had to be helped to assess the risk to themselves and those around them, enabling everyone to mitigate the risks while ensuring that the most vulnerable were protected, thereby minimizing the need for government-led interventions – indeed, being a bit more like Sweden.[16]

Of course, not everyone agreed with that, nor with the assessment that Sweden had been right all along. Within the Swedish scientific and medical community, debate about strategy had simmered and steamed, with a group – named the '22 researchers' – calling for tougher measures. Back in the spring they had published a blistering attack on the public health agency in an op-ed piece in *Dagens Nyheter*. Those putting their name to the article were from institutions across the country, including Lund University, the Karolinska Institute in Stockholm, Umeå University, Sahlgrenska University Hospital in Gothenburg, Danderyd Hospital in Stockholm, Gothenburg University, and Uppsala University.[17]

The piece had referred to the shocking toll on the most vulnerable, and to how the virus had free rein in nursing homes. The price of the country's hands-off approach had been too high, they stated, but although they were just saying what researchers across the world were saying, their criticism had not been welcomed, and some of them claimed to have been pilloried or reprimanded. Responding to the piece, Tegnell said that the twenty-two researchers had not been 'leaders in their field'. The group of twenty-two *forskare* would expand to include fifty scientists and another 150 supporting members, taking the name, Science Forum COVID-19. (*Vetenskapsforum COVID-19*) and continuing their criticism.[18]

Europe and the Second Wave – Second Lockdowns – EU Traffic Light System – ECDC Mapping – Regional Differences

By October, coronavirus cases were doubling across Europe every 9–10 days, and the continent had become gripped by a second wave of infection.

In many countries, the daily numbers of confirmed cases exceeded their spring peaks, but this was mostly because there had been a lot more testing; death rates were substantially lower. Most countries had failed to use the summer to build robust testing and contact-tracing operations, and so, come autumn and the second wave, they had to fall back on blunt measures such as closing down the hospitality sector (bars and pubs) and introducing quarantines and curfews.[19] Cities and regions again faced local lockdowns or other lesser restrictions – circuit breakers – and once more, countries introduced travel restrictions against each other.

Ireland had become the first EU member state to enter a new lockdown, imposing a six-week circuit breaker on 22 October. A spike in September left the country's test and trace system overwhelmed.[20]

Praised for a swift initial response to COVID-19 in the spring, by October Czechia had declared a state of emergency and was in second lockdown after recording thousands of new cases per day. On 22 October, the country recorded the highest per capita death rate in the world, and the worst infection rate in Europe. In addition, the deputy prime minister had announced that he had tested positive for coronavirus.

Others hard hit were the Netherlands and Belgium. The Netherlands, which dithered while cases rose steadily until they were higher than in Spain or France, returned to a partial lockdown. In Belgium, a night curfew was introduced, and Frank Vandenbroucke, the Belgian health minister, said that they could 'no longer control' what was happening, and that they were 'close to a tsunami'.[21] In France too, night curfews were introduced in Paris and several other cities, and the government was considering extending a national state of emergency to February 2021. In Dijon and Clermont, hospitals were reported to have cancelled non-COVID operations, with doctors saying that the new wave was already worse than the first. By the end of October, an overwhelmed France, and Germany, were set to impose renewed national lockdowns (lockdown 'light' in Germany, a partial lockdown). Curfews had been imposed in Berlin, Munich, Frankfurt-on-Main, Bremen, and Hamburg, and Munich had imposed a full lockdown.[22]

For its part, Spain had become the first European country to pass one million cases, reaching that milestone on 20–21 October.[23] The country had relaxed one of the world's longest lockdowns in May, but had struggled to contain new outbreaks. Madrid had accounted for around one third of the cases, and Spain was grappling with an underperforming test and contact-tracing system, a buckling healthcare system, and political quarrels that were impeding containment measures.[24]

In an attempt to limit the spread of COVID-19, EU member states had adopted a 'traffic light' system to maintain free movement within the bloc under safe conditions. Mapping would be published weekly by the ECDC, showing the risk levels across the regions of Europe and each level would be indicated using the colours 'red', 'orange', 'green', and 'grey'. The traffic light colour of a given region would depend on the number of new cases per 100,000 over the last fourteen days and the rate of positive cases. Using the map, members would decide what restrictions to put in place. The map would also provide travellers with general information as to the risk level at their destination.[25]

In the new traffic light system: 'red' would indicate high risk with more than 50 cases per 100,000 people (more than 500 per million), with 4 per cent positivity, or more than 150 cases per 100,000 (more than 1500 per million), with less than 4 per cent test positivity; 'orange' would indicate medium risk with more than 25 cases per 100,000 (more than 250 per million), with 4 per cent positivity, or between 25 and 150 cases per 100,000 (between 250 and 1500 per million), with less than 4 per cent positivity; 'green' would indicate low risk with less than 25 cases per 100,000 (less than 250 per million), with less than 4 per cent positivity. The fourth colour, 'grey', was provided for areas where there were insufficient data or where the number of tests carried out per 100,000 was considered too low.[26]

Almost every province and region in Europe showed up 'red' (high risk), but the mapping also showed up the 'successful' countries: Germany, Italy, and the Nordic countries.[27]

More specifically, ECDC mapping updated 22 October 2020, and informing the EU coordinated approach, showed as 'red' regions: the Iberian Peninsula, the Balearics, Malta, Corsica, Sardinia, Sicily, and the Italian peninsula apart from the tip of Calabria. Also 'red' were West Macedonia in Greece, Bulgaria, Romania, Croatia, Hungary, Slovenia, Austria, Liechtenstein, Slovakia, Czechia, Poland, Berlin, France, Luxembourg, the Netherlands, Region Stockholm, Iceland, and Ireland.[28]

In the mapping, the toe of Italy in Calabria, much of Greece, Cyprus, Germany excluding Berlin, and the Baltic States, were 'orange' regions. Also 'orange' countries and regions were Denmark, Sweden, excluding Region Stockholm, western Norway and areas around Oslo, and Troms and Finnmark in the north, and southern Finland.[29]

In Greece, the Peloponnese region, parts of the west, Crete, and East Macedonia and Thrace were 'green', as were central Norway and the rest of northern Norway, and Lapland and the rest of northern and eastern Finland.[30]

The UK, Belgium, and Liechtenstein were 'grey' areas, meaning that no or insufficient data were available. Switzerland and much of the Balkans were outside of the system.[31]

The mapping showed regional differences in the 14-day notification rate per 100,000 inhabitants. Mapping showed rates of more than 150 per 100,000 (1,500 per million) across: Spain, and the areas around Lisbon in Portugal; Malta; France and Corsica, Belgium, the Netherlands and Luxembourg; western, and parts of northern Italy; northern areas of Austria; Liechtenstein; Slovenia and Croatia; part of northern Greece; south-west Bulgaria; Romania; Slovakia; Czechia; Poland; Berlin; Region Stockholm; Iceland; Ireland; and, across all of the nations of the UK, including London, but excepting the rest of south-east England.[32]

It showed rates of between 50 and 149.9 per 100,000 (500 to 1,499 per million) in: Portugal; the Mediterranean regions of Castelon, Valencia, Alicante, and the Balearics, in Spain; eastern regions and parts of northern Italy and Sardinia and Sicily; Cyprus; southern Austria; parts of Hungary; small parts of Greece including Athens; much of Bulgaria; western and southern Germany, and Saxony; Latvia and Lithuania; the area around Helsinki and west-central Finland; Sweden; Sogn og Fjordane, and Hordaland in western Norway; Denmark; and, south-east England.[33]

The mapping showed rates of between 25 and 49.9 per 100,000 (250 to 499 per million) in: parts of Greece; eastern Germany and Schleswig-Holstein; Estonia; southern Finland, excluding Helsinki; and, parts of Nordland, Troms and Finnmark in northern Norway, Møre og Romsdal in western Norway, and the area around Oslo. Finally, it showed rates of less than 250 per million inhabitants in the rest of Norway, and across much of eastern and northern Finland; and parts of Greece.[34]

The differing rates of coronavirus and the patchwork of incidence across the continent brought differing restrictions within individual countries – the UK had tier systems across its four nations – and, with that, added difficulty for governments and health agencies in keeping 'confused' populations engaged with the measures. Governments needed to keep their populations on side and ensure compliance and consent – adherence was key – especially as it looked as though measures of varying degree would have to be in place for some time to come. Indeed, Angela Merkel had given warning of 'a long hard winter ahead'.[35]

From the Commission in Brussels, von der Leyen offered a similar sober message, saying after a video conference of EU leaders that the spread of the virus would overwhelm healthcare systems if urgent action was not taken. EUR 220 million had been made available to move COVID-19 patients across borders to prevent hospitals being overwhelmed.[36]

Earlier in October, Carlson had said that any measures introduced in Sweden to combat a rise in infection – probably at a local or regional level – would likely remain in place for some time to come, perhaps for another year.[37]

Another bleak message came from the UK, albeit in a leaked report obtained by *The Spectator* magazine. A worst-case scenario could see a second wave across the UK far greater than the first and dragging on until March or April 2021.[38]

By end-October, the mapping showed almost the entire continent of Europe as 'red', and lockdowns to some degree or another – increased measures, lockdown-light – had been applied in England, France, Belgium, Germany, Italy, and Greece.

By mid-November, all of mainland Europe was 'red', as was Cyprus, Malta, Madeira, and the Azores. Only Ireland, Iceland, the least populous parts of Norway, and most of Finland, were 'orange'. Greenland and western parts of Finland were green. Switzerland and much of the Balkans were outside of the system.[39]

Sweden and the Second Wave

The term 'second wave' had been used by scientists, governments, experts, and the media – especially the media – to refer to a resurgence in coronavirus cases, following the initial peak, and then fall. However, there was no fixed definition of what constituted a 'second wave' in epidemiology. There was no threshold that new daily cases or infection rate had to cross.[40]

The ECDC had explained that the term, 'second wave', was used mostly in descriptions of influenza, and that it had become a much-discussed concept because the 1918 flu pandemic saw a mutation of the virus between 'waves' and became more dangerous, bringing many more deaths. Talk of 'waves' in relation to the 2019 coronavirus had circulated in the media – a lot – but what epidemiologists referred to in the current pandemic, was a resurgence of cases, and not a new 'wave'.[41]

Nevertheless, if using the widespread (though epidemiologically inaccurate) definition of a 'second wave' as a rise in cases after a period of falling numbers, then it was indeed the case that Sweden, along with many other European countries in the autumn, had experienced a second wave. In the USA though, a 'second wave' might not be seen at all because the country remained in its first, whereas in countries such as Poland and Czechia, which had recorded many cases in the autumn, there had been no experience of a 'first wave'.[42]

While Sweden had not been experiencing the second wave to the same extent as the UK, France, and Spain, Tegnell had warned that the country's infection rate was heading in the wrong direction. Cases were creeping up perhaps because offices had become busier again, and because shopping and going out had gone back to normal levels (in Region Stockholm cases in September had quadrupled, and across Sweden in early-October the number of patients receiving intensive care had doubled). After eight of Sweden's regions reported outbreaks of the virus linked to universities, the minister for higher education, Matilda Ernkrans, told students that unfortunately there were 'far too many' of them not taking responsibility (she was referring to student parties) and that they had to 'get a grip now'.[43]

The Swedish strategy for a second wave had converged with that of Germany, entailing rapid large-scale testing and contact-tracing to identify and supress outbreaks early. When someone did test positive, their entire household had to go into quarantine lasting five to seven days (in comparison to two weeks in other countries). Apparently, the risk of spreading COVID-19 in a second week was small and shrinking. Other contacts were alerted that they might be infected, urged to work from home for a week, and to get tested if they showed even the slightest of symptoms over the next two weeks, taking care not to see elderly relatives. Schoolchildren were exempt, the government believing that any gain from shutting them away was far outweighed by the harm done to their education.[44]

While the WHO had advised against quarantine of less than two weeks, the Swedish approach was to have measures that people could live with for at least a year given that the virus was going to be present for a long time. The aim was to stop as much transmission as possible without unduly disrupting people's lives, especially in ways that harmed mental health (and extended isolation was a growing harm to mental health). Sweden was a high-trust society where people followed the rules, but asking too much of them would lower compliance and thus spread the disease.[45]

Disruption to people's lives, damaged mental health, and subsequent stress deserved consideration. Stress caused by extended isolation or by other risk factors could lead to suicide. Studies had shown that during major disasters there were 'fewer' suicides, but as the effects of post-traumatic stress disorders began to play out, there were 'more'. This seemed to have happened during the COVID-19 pandemic. In the early months, many countries reported fewer cases, but a 2022 review of 1,052 studies of suicide found that most of the studies reported an increasing number during the pandemic. In Sweden though, there had been no increase, but rather a small decrease from 2019 to 2021.[46]

Additionally, extended isolation during lockdown where couples had been forced to remain under the same roof, 'cabin fever' perhaps – talking frivolously – could lead to increased cases of domestic abuse. A study of the USA and six other countries had concluded that lockdowns increased domestic abuse by around 8 per cent. Although Sweden had not been one of the seven countries analyzed in the study, the reported number of cases of abuse against women and girls by a present or former partner had declined by around 25 per cent between 2020 and 2022.[47]

By the end of October 2020, the regions of Uppsala, Skåne, Stockholm, Västra Götaland, and Östergötland, had introduced stricter coronavirus measures following an increase in patients in hospital and in elderly care, and an increase in positive tests. These regions included some of Sweden's largest cities and towns: Stockholm, Gothenburg, Malmö, Uppsala, Linköping, Helsingborg, Norrköping, and Lund, and accounting for more than 3,000,000 people, and approaching a third of the population. The measures which were described by the public health agency as 'general recommendations' included: avoidance of indoor environments such as shops, shopping centres, museums, libraries, swimming pools and gyms; avoidance of concerts, performances, sports training (excluding children under the age of 15), matches, and competitions; and avoidance of physical contact with people other than those lived with, including the holding of parties and other similar social gatherings. While the government had previously okayed the raising to 300 the limit on attendees at public events, the regions introducing stricter measures were keeping the limit at 50.[48] Into November, another five regions introduced tighter measures – Region Halland, Region Jönköping, Region Örebro, Region Kronoberg, and Region Södermanland – joining the earlier five regions and including a new roll-call of Swedish cities and towns such as Halmstad, Jönköping, Örebro, Växjö, Eskilstuna, and Nyköping, and covering over half of the Swedish population in ten out of twenty-one regions. The remaining eleven regions were less densely populated, with a low level of spread of the virus, though Region Västmanland (including the sizeable town of Västerås) was mulling over the introduction of local measures.

Businesses had been urged to take measures to reduce the risk of spreading infection including reducing the number of customers in shops. The importance of working from home was emphasised by Tegnell, as workplaces had become a key source of new infections. Both employers and employees had been asked to do their best to make it possible to work from home as much as possible.[49]

Well into autumn 2020 though, Sweden remained one of the only countries in the world that still did not recommend mask-wearing. It had been argued that they provided a false sense of security that undermined social distancing efforts. However, it was recognized that they could play a part in fighting local or regional outbreaks, particularly on public transport where face-coverings could be beneficial. Indeed, impetus for wearing them was expected to come from the commercial and industrial sectors as firms emulated the decision taken by Swedish telecom giant, Ericsson, to make mask-wearing compulsory for employees and visitors to their offices.[50] In late-summer, the Karolinska had recommend mask-wearing to its teaching staff and students on their return to campus.

As the second wave gripped Europe, Tegnell continued to defend his stance on mask-wearing. Countries such as France which had obligatory face-covering in place, or mask-wearing, had still experienced a big spread of the disease.[51]

Although Tegnell, the public health agency, and the government, were reluctant to bring in even stricter measures despite the upward trend – full lockdown, say – it seemed possible that they would have no choice. If the trajectory continued and led to more cases of serious illness requiring intensive care, a spike in deaths, and an overwhelmed healthcare system, then even stricter measures would have to be introduced. Sweden could be on the same path as the UK and France towards replacing tiered or regional measures with a national lockdown. But wasn't a large part of the country already shutting down through the introduction of local restrictions across almost half its regions?[52]

Sweden's 6,000 Death Toll – Löfven in Self-Isolation – Mutated Coronavirus in Danish Mink – Risk to Vaccines

As Sweden's coronavirus death toll passed the new and grim milestone of 6,000 on 6 November, Stefan Löfven shared on social media that he and his wife – Ulla – had gone into self-isolation after a person close to him came into contact with another individual with confirmed COVID-19.[53]

They themselves had no symptoms but the prime minister said that he would work remotely, and that in accordance with the health recommendations they would be taking the required tests as soon as possible. He also took the opportunity to urge Swedes to follow the guidelines of the public health agency. Löfven had generally worked remotely anyway.[54]

Meanwhile, in Denmark and in Sweden, there had been an escalation in an outbreak of a mutated form of coronavirus in mink farms. In Sweden, the virus had first been identified in a mink herd in Sölvesborg, Region Blekinge – southern Sweden – in October. Infected mink had also been found in the Netherlands and Spain, but the outbreak had been spreading particularly fast in Denmark with over 200 farms in Jutland having been affected. After a report from the SSI that the mutated virus had been transmitted to humans and had infected several people already, a cull of every one of Denmark's 17 million mink was planned. Frederiksen, the prime minister, had described the situation as 'very, very serious', saying that the mutated virus would pose a risk to the effectiveness of a future COVID-19 vaccine. Denmark had been the world's biggest producer of mink fur, with over 1,000 breeders, and China and Hong Kong were the industry's principal export markets. During the cull, the fur, or animal pelts, would also be destroyed.[55] In July, after an outbreak at a mink farm in the Aragón province of Spain, 100,000 animals were culled. In the Netherlands, tens of thousands of animals had been slaughtered.[56]

In response to the Danish situation, sampling had been carried out among all the herds in Sweden (there were about forty mink farms), and the Swedish Board of Agriculture (*Jordbruksverket*) stated that the infection had been confined to mink farms in Blekinge itself. Herds had been subjected to restrictions, even those that were uninfected. Animals were not allowed to be moved, tools and equipment were not to be shared, and hygiene regimes were to be followed. Farms were not to receive any visitors, for it had been people who had introduced the coronavirus to mink in the first place, observed Karl Ståhl, the state veterinary epidemiologist at the National Veterinary Institute, SVA (*Statens Veterinärmedicinska Anstalt, SVA*).[57]

While Sweden had not planned to cull its animals, the annual pelting had been due to take place in November anyway, with all but the breeding stock graded and slaughtered, and the pelts prepared for export (Denmark's loss was Sweden's gain). Ståhl said that some 80 per cent of Sweden's farmed mink would be killed in coming weeks. Nevertheless, developments in Denmark would be followed closely, and there was great concern among breeders in Sweden about both the infection and the consequences in Denmark.[58]

Meanwhile, in Denmark, bars, restaurants, public transport, and all public indoor sports were closed, shut down, or cancelled across North Jutland.[59] 'The eyes of the world' were on Denmark, said Frederiksen, though she might have wanted to add that the world's eyes had shifted from Sweden.

In addition to pigs, camels, bats, and cats already mentioned as being among the more than sixty mammal species known to be susceptible to coronavirus, gorillas and chimpanzees, foxes, yaks, giant pandas, and koalas were also susceptible. Whales, dolphins, and seals might be too. Virologists had expressed concern about 'reverse spillover', which is the passing on of the virus from humans to domestic and wild animals. This brought risk of animals becoming a new reservoir of the disease – and passing it back to humans ironically – making it more difficult to control. The risk of the virus mutating into another novel coronavirus was always present.[60]

Several mutant versions of the virus had been found in mink, according to SSI, and some of the mutations were in the spike protein which is significant in the body's immune system, and a key target for vaccines. The WHO had urged calm and said that researchers should wait before reaching any conclusion on whether the mutation would affect vaccines. There had been no indication that it would.[61]

In the event, days after announcing that the mutations could jeopardise the effectiveness of potential COVID-19 vaccines, scientists had reviewed the data and said that the mutations themselves were not particularly concerning because there was little evidence that they allowed the virus to spread more easily among people, make it more deadly, or would jeopardise therapeutics and vaccines. Nevertheless, culling the mink had probably been necessary given the rapid and uncontrolled spread among the animals, which made them a massive viral source that could easily infect people (there had been approximately three times more mink than people in Denmark).[62]

After the Danish cull, there had been too many bodies to incinerate at once and so shallow mass graves had been dug at a military site in western Jutland. In December, it was reported that groundwater in the area was feared to have become contaminated.[63]

In early-2021, mink breeding was banned in Sweden throughout the rest of 2021. The SVA – veterinary institute – had said that evidence from Denmark and the Netherlands showed that while the virus was still spreading in the community it was difficult to stop it from being introduced to the mink population. Under those conditions it was not considered appropriate from an infection control perspective to continue increasing the mink population in the country. Farmers could keep their animals so that operations could begin 2022, but any pups born before then would have to be put down.[64]

Statistics, October–November 2020 – On-Going European Toll – Tighter Measures in Sweden

Into autumn, the virus continued its grip on the continent and according to data compiled by Johns Hopkins University, at end-October close to 10 million confirmed cases and more than 260,000 fatalities had been recorded across

Europe since the pandemic began. Across the world there had been more than 46 million confirmed cases and 1.25 million deaths, with a handful of countries accounting for three-quarters of those deaths: the USA, Brazil, India, Mexico, Peru, the UK, and Italy. Three of them – the USA, Brazil, and India – had accounted for half the world's deaths.[65]

Since the start of the coronavirus outbreak, cumulative deaths across the Nordic countries by end-October had been recorded as: in Sweden 5,938, Denmark 721, Finland 358, Norway 282, and Iceland 12. The death toll in Iceland had been static at 10 since 21 April, but the 11th death had been recorded by 16 October, and the 12th death by 28 October.[66]

In the rest of Europe, the UK, Italy, France, and Spain had recorded the highest number of cumulative deaths by end-October. In the UK, the figure was 46,645, Italy 38,618, France 36,827, and Spain 35,878.[67]

Across Europe on the measure of daily new confirmed deaths per million (on a rolling seven-day average) at end-October, Czechia had recorded 15.64, Andorra 11.08, Belgium 10.91, Montenegro 8.64, Liechtenstein 7.47, Slovenia 7.08, and Bosnia and Herzegovina 6.96, followed by Hungary, Romania, Poland, Switzerland, France, Moldova, Croatia, then Bulgaria above 4. Then the UK, the EU taken together, Spain, Italy, Malta, and Europe taken together above 3, followed by Portugal, Luxembourg, Austria, and Russia above 2. As for the Nordic countries, Denmark recorded 0.52 cases on that metric, Iceland 0.42, Finland 0.13, Norway 0.08, and Sweden 0.07.[68]

Across Europe on the measure of daily new cases per million (on a rolling seven-day average) at end-October, Belgium had recorded 1,520.44 cases, Andorra 1,326, Czechia 1,122.99, Luxembourg 963.84, and Slovenia 895.67, followed by Switzerland, Liechtenstein, France, San Marino, Croatia, Slovakia, Poland, Bosnia and Herzegovina, Spain, Austria, the EU, and Italy above 413. The UK had recorded 330.4, while among the Nordic countries it was Iceland that had recorded the highest number of daily new cases with 195.96, next came Sweden with 193.49, then Denmark with 170.54, Norway 67.49, and Finland 37.62.[69]

Over 10–11 November, the UK became the first country in Europe to record over 50,000 cumulative deaths, recording 49,861 on 10 November and 50,457 on 11 November. On those dates, Italy, France, and Spain – countries with the next highest death rates in Europe – were still some-way behind. The UK had become the sixth country in the world to pass 50,000 deaths, the first five reaching that figure being, the USA, Brazil, India, Mexico, and then Peru. The entire continent of Africa had recorded only just over 46,000 COVID-19 deaths on 11 November.[70] Over 16–17 November, the USA became the first country in the world to record over 250,000 cumulative deaths, recording 248,348 on 16 November and 250,057 on 17 November.[71]

Meanwhile, another three Swedish regions had introduced tighter measures – Region Kalmar County, Region Norbotten, and Region Västerbotten – joining the earlier ten (but now including less densely populated areas of the country) and a continuing roll-call of Sweden's towns – large and small – and including Kalmar, Västervik, Oskarshamn, Luleå, Piteå, Boden, Kiruna, Umeå, and Skellefteå. Thirteen of Sweden's 21 regions were now subject to stricter restrictions issued by the public health agency. In addition, Region Blekinge in the south, bordering Skåne and Kalmar, and including the city of Karlskrona, had introduced its own recommendations to be followed alongside the national recommendations.[72]

In a response to what had been seen as an 'environment of risk', the government proposed that the sale of alcohol should be stopped after 22.00 in restaurants, nightclubs, pubs, and bars, and that venues licenced to sell alcohol must close at 22.30. People were becoming too relaxed when it came to following coronavirus recommendations, lowering their guard. Lena Hallengren, the health and social affairs minister, said that she understood that people were tired, and that they were missing their regular lives, but the situation right now was 'unsustainable'. The pandemic would 'require more sacrifices from us all, not fewer'.[73]

Offsetting that bad news, optimistic signals had come from the Stockholm-based ECDC. The head of the agency had said that the first vaccinations against COVID-19 could be underway in the first quarter of 2021. This was the vaccine developed by US pharmaceutical giant Pfizer Inc. and BioNTech SE of Germany, which could be authorised for use across the EU early in the new year.[74]

The number of people testing positive for coronavirus continued to increase, putting greater pressure on the healthcare system. With community spread across most parts of Sweden, another four regions became subject to the stricter restrictions issued by public health agency. These were: Region Dalarna, Gotland Municipality, Region Värmland, and Region Västmanland. and included the towns and cities of: Borlänge, Falun, Visby, Karlstad, Kristenhamn, and Västerås. Another three regions swiftly followed – Region Gävleborg, Region Västernorrland, and Region Jämtland Härjedalen, including the towns of Gävle, Sandviken, Sundsvall, Östersund, and Strömsund – so that by just after mid-November twenty of the twenty-one regions had been subjected to stricter restrictions recommended by the public health agency. The remaining one was Region Blekinge which had applied its own recommendations.

With the entire country under stricter measures – Sweden and almost the entire map of Europe was coloured 'red' on the EU traffic light system – a ban on public events of more than eight people was put in place. In March, the limit had been set at 50, and although it had been raised to 300 for specific events in late-October, none of the regions chose to implement that new higher limit. Now, in November, all regions agreed on an audience limit of eight. Workplaces were not affected by the ban, but the public health agency recommendation remained the same. People should work from home as much as possible. The limit of eight for public gatherings should also be the norm for private gatherings such as dinners, parties, and visits to gyms and the like. Across most regions too, recommendations asked that people refrain from close contact with those from other households, and non-essential visits to indoor environments such as shops, gyms, and museums. Government ministers also urged people not to look for loopholes or justifications to continue doing these things.[75] By 20 November, Stockholm and Malmö had followed the lead of Gothenburg and announced the closure of public swimming pools, museums, art galleries, gyms, and other municipal meeting places. Instead, people were urged to take exercise outside.[76]

As regards the avoidance of close contact with others – social or physical distancing – it was inevitable that once again the matter of mask-wearing came to the fore in November. While Michael Ryan from the WHO Health Emergencies Programme had said that in the spring there had been 'very high compliance' with voluntary measures in Sweden, and that the high proportion of single-person households had been an advantage, the country had faced 'difficulties'. He advised that WHO advice on mask-wearing was clear. They worked. The issue of face-coverings, of course, had been repeatedly raised with the public health agency by both Swedish and foreign journalists alike. Löfven had pointed out that there was no recommendation against wearing masks, while Carlson said that they were focussing on the prevention of crowding rather than advising on mask-wearing in such situations. Answers from neither were given on whether masks should be worn in situations where crowding could not be avoided.[77]

Pressure on the public health agency over mask-wearing was also coming from the Royal Swedish Academy of Sciences (*Kungliga Vetenskapsakademien, KVA*). Its COVID-19 expert group had concluded that good ventilation and the use of masks were important measures in reducing the spread of infection in indoor spaces and on public transport. There was new experimental and epidemiological evidence that mask-wearing reduced the risk of airborne transmission, and none that it might have the opposite effect, said Staffan Normark, chair of the KVA expert group, and professor of molecular microbiology and infection control at the Karolinska Institute. While it was important to follow the recommendations of the public health agency, all the tools in the toolbox – including mask-wearing or face-coverings – were required to bring down the rate of infection.[78]

Löfven, Address to the Nation, November 2020 – COVID-19 and the Swedish Royals

On 22 November, Löfven delivered a new address to the nation, eight months after the one made in the spring – in March – and in which he had told Swedes that the next few months would 'be stressful'.

Now, in November, it was clear, he said, that it would 'be some time' before the country could 'return to what we consider normal'. The short respite that had been experienced during the summer and autumn was truly over, and now, once again, he was asking for something that was very difficult but completely necessary. People's health and lives were still at risk, and the danger was increasing. More and more people were being infected, more ICU beds were being used to treat seriously ill COVID-19 patients, and more and more were dying.[79]

In the spring, he said, the country had managed to 'flatten the curve of transmission' as people took responsibility and gave overworked health and social care personnel a chance to cope with the acute crisis. In the autumn, too many people had neglected to follow the advice and recommendations, but now – as Advent and (*Luciadagen*) St Lucia Day, 13 December, approached – they were again starting to take responsibility. Fewer people were travelling, and more were working from home. Even so, 'we must all do more', Löfven said.[80]

He went on to highlight what everyone should do. In addition to keeping distance, working from home if possible, and washing hands frequently, they should: stay updated as to the advice and recommendations; only get together with those in the household; if living alone, choose no more than one or two friends to socialize with; and stay at home if displaying the slightest symptoms. Everything that was unnecessary ought to be cancelled, re-booked, or postponed.[81]

Although it would be some time before the coronavirus crisis was over, until it was, this would be the 'new normal' for all of Sweden. Although everything might seem dark just now, the situation he said was 'not hopeless'. Sweden was being tested, but it would pull through, and despite everything the health and social care systems were functioning. We all had to take the situation very seriously, and 'do so with discipline, determination and courage'. We must show our solidarity and our sense of responsibility. These were stronger than the virus that would be defeated, he said.[82]

Towards the end of November, it had been reported that two members of the royal family had tested positive for COVID-19 – the king's son, prince Carl Philip, and his wife, princess Sofia. Both had experienced mild flu-like symptoms though felt well under the circumstances, and had gone into quarantine with their two sons, Alexander, and Gabriel (their third child, Julian, would be born in 2021). Contact-tracing had been carried out, with the king, queen, crown princess and her husband all testing negative. They had all been in close contact with each other a few days earlier at the private funeral for the queen's brother, Walter Sommerlath, who had died at the Karolinska in October.[83]

Sweden Just Like the Rest of Scandinavia

As the second wave of coronavirus swept across Europe, and as all of Sweden's regions introduced stricter restrictions based on public health agency recommendations, there now seemed to be more that united the approaches taken by the different Scandinavian countries than which divided them.[84]

Sweden's earlier light touch approach had contrasted markedly with the swift lockdowns that had brought Denmark, Norway, and Finland to a halt. Now, in the second wave, the Swedish approach had taught the other Nordic countries that they did not have to go into lockdown and had shown them where to be more careful. Following the example set by Sweden earlier – and the Swedish data gathered – schools had been kept open during the second wave. Keeping them open did not contribute to spreading coronavirus. Society could remain open, other than for some restrictions on how many people could gather, and early closing for hospitality and entertainment venues.[85]

In applying stricter guidelines – save for formally advising on the use of face-coverings – Sweden too had undergone a learning experience. There had been evidence that the more restrictive approaches in the rest of Scandinavia had worked better and did not have the feared destructive effect on the economy.[86]

While there was no arguing with the high Swedish death toll in comparison to other Scandinavian countries, Sweden and its neighbours had avoided the alarming rates of infection and deaths suffered in the rest of Europe. Had this been because Scandinavians tended to trust politicians and authorities, and were willing to obey rules? Was the entire Nordic region now benefiting from decades of social democracy, and Europe's highest levels of trust in government?[87]

While a study conducted by the European Commission showed that Denmark and Finland had the highest levels of trust in government, in Sweden too – in spite of a dip in June because of the mounting death toll – trust in authorities also remained high.[88] That said though, given the tenor of the prime minister's address to the nation in November, perhaps trust was wearing a little thin and people's behaviour was reflecting this, or perhaps people were simply wearying a little.

Deadliest November Since 1918

Based on COVID-19 cases reported between late-summer and mid-autumn, and on how the virus might spread until the following spring, at the end of November the public health agency suggested that the coronavirus outbreak would peak in mid-December.

Carlson stressed that this could change as the situation developed, and that the actual outcome would depend on several factors. The scenario had been presented to help other Swedish authorities organize their own coronavirus contingency plans. Although the peak would come mid-December, that did not mean that the virus would go away any time soon. Indeed, the scenario as presented suggested that the spread of infection would remain higher than in summer and continue right through to late-February 2021.[89]

Since the start of the coronavirus outbreak, cumulative deaths across the Nordic countries by end-November had been recorded as: in Sweden 6,681, Denmark 837, Finland 399, Norway 332, and in Iceland 26.[90]

According to Statistics Sweden, more deaths had been registered in November 2020 (8,088 deaths from all causes) than in any other November in more than hundred years. In 1918, during the year that 'Spanish flu' broke out, there had been 16,600 deaths from all causes that month.[91]

In the rest of Europe in 2020, the UK, Italy, France, and Spain had recorded the highest number of cumulative deaths by end-November. In the UK, the figure was 58,545, Italy 55,576, France 52,818, and Spain 45,069.[92]

Across Europe on the measure of daily new confirmed deaths per million (on a rolling seven-day average) at end-November, Slovenia had recorded 23.23, Bulgaria 20.01, Liechtenstein 14.98, Bosnia and Herzegovina 14.84, Hungary 13.82, Croatia 13.58, and Poland 12.76, followed by Montenegro, Macedonia 14.88, Bosnia and Herzegovina 14.76, Hungary 13.78, followed by Croatia, Poland, Montenegro, Czechia, Italy, Austria, Belgium, Luxembourg, Switzerland, and Greece each above 9. The UK had recorded 6.74 on the measure, the EU taken together 7.98, and Europe as a whole 6.64. As for the Nordic countries, Sweden recorded 3.87, Denmark 1.18, Norway 0.55, Finland 0.39, and Iceland 0.[93]

On the measure of daily new cases per million (on a rolling seven-day average) across Europe at end-November, Serbia had recorded 1,023.91 cases, Montenegro 829.55, Andorra 814.44, Luxembourg 802.71, Croatia 796.28, and San Marino 760.28, followed by Lithuania, Slovenia, Hungary, and Austria above 500. The UK had recorded 214.61, and among the Nordic countries it was Sweden that had the highest number of daily new cases with 489.78, next came Denmark with 216.92, then Norway 77.55, Finland 76.63, and Iceland 42.85.[94]

Over 2–3 December the UK passed the milestone of 60,000 cumulative deaths from COVID-19, and Italy and France had not been that far behind with a toll of well over 50,000 in each country. Next came Spain then Russia which had recorded over 40,000 deaths each.[95]

Vaccine Approval – Plans for Rollout

After China had shared publicly the genetic sequence of the novel coronavirus back in January 2020, urgent work began in pharmaceutical laboratories all over the world to develop a vaccine to counter it.

Earlier research to develop a vaccine against SARS and MERS had already established a body of knowledge about the structure and workings of coronaviruses, and this accelerated the research to develop a vaccine against COVID-19. By November 2020 positive results had been announced by several laboratories after analysis of vaccine trials. These included candidate vaccines developed by: Pfizer/BioNTech, USA and Germany; University of Oxford/AstraZeneca, UK and Sweden; Sinopharm, China; Sinovac, China; CanSinoBio, China; CoronaVac, China; Gam-COVID-Vac (Sputnik V), Russia; Moderna/NIAID/others, USA; and, Janssen Pharmaceuticals (Johnson & Johnson), Belgium. There were many others too, including candidates developed in India. What would normally take up to ten years to develop, had taken mere months.

To end the crisis, it was not just a case of developing COVID-19 vaccines, everyone in the world had to have fair and equitable access to diagnostics and treatments, and one of the pillars of ACT-A (the Access to COVID-19 Tools Accelerator) was COVAX. Back in September 2020, just as the world had seen the one millionth death from COVID-19, the UN had welcomed nearly US$ 1 billion in pledges to bolster access to tests, treatments, and vaccines, to end COVID-19. Among those commitments was US$ 10 million (SEK 89.4 million) from Sweden to COVAX and to the support of low- and middle-income countries and their access to vaccines.[96] In spite of scepticism around the vaccines produced by Russia, China, and India, African countries were turning towards them because the vaccines produced in the west and which were to be made available (the COVAX facility through GAVI, and ACT Accelerator) seemed unlikely to be acquired early enough to control the second wave being recorded across the continent into January 2021.

For Sweden itself, the government had decided to take part in the EU's joint procurement of vaccines, and by the end of November 2020 several EU/EEA countries including Sweden had published interim recommendations for vaccine deployment to 'first priority' groups. Elderly people over 70 would be prioritized, as would adults with co-morbidities (people with two or more medical conditions), healthcare and social care workers, and other workers at risk including those in essential public services. Vaccinations would be delivered at dedicated vaccination centres and at healthcare centres.[97]

In Sweden, an electronic immunisation registry system was already in place, and work was ongoing for the adaptation – legal as well as IT adaptation – of the national vaccination register for registration of all vaccinations against COVID-19.[98]

Some 2.6 million people would be prioritized under the categories described earlier, and the vaccines to protect them were to be available just as soon as they had been approved for use by the relevant Swedish agencies, and in accordance with established routines. It had been expected that vaccinations would begin in Sweden sometime in January 2021, at the earliest (they actually started on 27 December 2020).[99] Headquartered in Amsterdam, the European Medicines Agency (EMA) was the body in charge of approving vaccines in the EU. Once it approved the Pfizer/BioNTech vaccine which had been placed before it, the planned first doses were expected to arrive in Sweden by Christmas, and into January up to 350,000 would have arrived.[100]

On 8 December 2020, the first person in the western world to receive a vaccination against coronavirus – outside of a trial – was a 90-year-old woman at the University Hospital Coventry, in England. She had received her first dose of the Pfizer/BioNTech vaccine which had been given regulatory approval in the UK only a few days before. Still a member of the EMA during the eleven-month transition period after 'Brexit', the UK had been able to give regulatory approval and begin vaccination because, under EU law, countries could invoke emergency powers to temporarily approve a vaccine in the event of a pandemic.[101] The second vaccine to be given regulatory approval in the UK was the Oxford/AstraZeneca vaccine at the end of December 2020. In January 2021, the Moderna vaccine was given UK regulatory approval. By way of contrast, in November, in China, Sinopharm was said to have vaccinated around 1 million people as part of an emergency-use programme (large-scale human testing outside clinical trials).[102]

As December had gotten underway, and Swedish 'advent candles' began to be lit, and *Luciadagen* was eagerly anticipated, it was reported by the National Board of Health and Welfare (*Socialstyrelsen*) that for the first time since spring, more than half of Sweden's intensive care unit patients were being treated for COVID-19. While 28 per cent of ICU beds were still available, every one of Sweden's twenty-one regions currently had COVID-19 patients in intensive care.[103] A week later, in Region Stockholm, ICU units had reportedly reached 99 per cent capacity for the first time during the pandemic. The region's healthcare workers had become so overworked that formal requests for help had gone out to other regions and to private health institutions for any available staff.[104] The request call for help had also gone out to the armed forces for the provision of doctors and medical equipment. It had been a lack of trained staff that was limiting the number of intensive care beds that could be used.[105]

Schools Break Up for Christmas

Into December, the number of those testing positive to coronavirus had continued to rise, and this was met with new measures.

In a joint press conference on 3 December, Löfven, Carlson, and Ekström, the education minister, announced that upper secondary schools (for over-16s) would be closed to students from the following week until after Christmas (they had previously been closed from mid-March to mid-June). This measure – intended to put a brake on the spread of infection and recommended by the public health agency – would see students switch to online distance learning for the remainder of the semester. If necessary, exceptions would be made for practical modules that couldn't be postponed, exams that couldn't be conducted online, teaching of students with special needs, and for students taking introductory language classes.[106]

The prime minister reminded Sweden's school students that they were trusted to be wise, and to understand that they were not on extended *jullov* (Christmas break) with the go-ahead for partying with friends. They were still 'in school' and should study, and he wanted parents to speak to them about the importance of following the recommendations.[107] Over a week later, Region Stockholm announced that it was recommending the closure of lower secondary schools (attended by students aged thirteen to fifteen years old) and a shift to online distance learning similar to the arrangements for older peers. The amount of contact between students had to be dramatically reduced, including socializing outside the home setting. Primary schools in Malmö had also come to an early close.[108]

In a further press conference on 8 December, just as the stricter regional recommendations were set to expire and to be replaced with national guidelines, Carlson warned that the outbreak might peak before or during Christmas. The situation continued to be serious for the country and there remained significant spread of infection with a great risk of spread over the Christmas break, which could end very badly. Unnecessary risks over Christmas would not be worth it.[109]

The ban on public gatherings of more than eight people would remain in place, and Swedes should stay in their current bubbles of social contacts, he said. Löfven reiterated that eight was also meant to set the standard for all private social gatherings. New contacts should be avoided, and as few people should be met as possible, and only briefly and at a distance, preferably outside.[110]

Travelling by train and bus was to be avoided, though if they had to travel – for example to parents and grandparents – they should do it responsibly and with bookable seats. Those visiting isolated elderly relations had to start social distancing measures around 10-days in advance of seeing anyone outside their usual social bubble.[111]

Later in the month, in a new round of measures, the prime minister announced that face-coverings would be recommended on public transport at certain times – rush hours, in effect. In attendance at this later press conference, on 18 December, Carlson stated that while masks did make a difference where social distance could not be maintained, they could hamper efforts to contain the disease where they replaced social distancing. It was not a general recommendation in Sweden that face-coverings be used either indoors or outdoors.[112]

Guidelines about the use of face-coverings were presented just before people returned to work after the Christmas break, but months after similar requirements had been announced in most other countries. Issued by the public health agency, the new recommendations stated that from 7 January 2021, and for those born 2004 or earlier – those over sixteen years of age – masks should be worn when travelling on public transport on weekdays, 07.00 to 09.00, and 16.00 to 18.00. For those passengers who did not have their own masks, public transport operators were recommended to provide them, and to inform how and when to wear them.[113]

Alpha-Variant of COVID-19 – First Vaccinations in Sweden and EU

Earlier, in the UK, just before the planned relaxation of coronavirus rules to allow households and families to mix over Christmas, a much more contagious variant of the virus had emerged – the Alpha-variant – and was affecting large parts of south-east England, including London. According to the WHO which had been in close contact with UK officials, the same mutation of COVID-19 had been detected in the Netherlands, Denmark, and Australia. Although the variation spread more rapidly than the original version, it had not been thought to be more deadly. In response, Ireland, France, Belgium, the Netherlands, Germany, and Italy announced the curtailment of flights and travel from the UK.[114] France halted all passenger, rail, freight, and ferry services across the Channel with thousands of trucks and other vehicles trapped in the UK. Until a testing process could be put in place, their occupants had to stay where they were in queues and allocated spaces in truck parks, unable to make it home in time for Christmas.

With the new Alpha-variant perhaps up to 70 per cent more transmissible than the original version, and with the likelihood of things becoming 'a lot worse' according to Professor Chris Whitty, chief medical officer for England, the plans to relax the rules over Christmas for up to five days had been scrapped.[115] By 26 December, cases of the Alpha-variant linked to people arriving from the UK had been identified in Spain, Switzerland, Sweden, and France. Cases had also been confirmed in Canada and Japan.[116]

Meanwhile, on 22 December the EU medicines regulator, the EMA, had recommended the Pfizer/BioNTech coronavirus vaccine for use across the EU27. Soon after the EMA decision, the EU Commission gave its approval for the use of the vaccine among 446 million inhabitants and a coordinated start to distribution and vaccination was set to begin on 27 December.[117] Although, Germany, Slovakia, and Hungary had begun administering vaccinations as soon as they had received shipments – saying they were not prepared to wait – the EU vaccine rollout began, said von der Leyen, in a 'touching moment of unity'. The first EU citizen to receive the vaccine was a 101-year-old woman, a care home resident from Halberstadt in Saxony-Anhalt, Germany.[118] The European rollout was also underway in Denmark, Czechia, Italy, and Spain. Beyond the EU, Israel also began vaccinations, hoping to give cover to one quarter of the population within a month.[119] On 6 January 2021 as the Pfizer/BioNTech vaccine was being rolled out across the EU, the EMA announced that it had given approval to the Moderna vaccine as well.

As anticipated, the planned first vaccinations had been given on 27 December in Sweden too, starting on a small scale in care homes and nursing homes, and among those receiving care at home, among other vulnerable groups, and for healthcare staff working with these groups. In total, Sweden had received 9,750 vaccine doses distributed across all twenty-one regions running the healthcare system. The first person to be vaccinated was 91-year-old Gunn-Britt Johnsson at a care home in Mjölby, Östergötland. Throughout the day, other regions around the country started their programmes too. A health centre in Råå, on the edge of Helsingborg, and a nursing home in Helsingborg itself, were the first in Region Skåne to begin the rollout. In Gothenburg in the west of Sweden, 99-year-old Rosa Johansson was the first to be vaccinated. From the first week in January, 80,000 doses were expected each week, and the goal was to offer vaccinations to the entire adult population by the first half of 2021. Löfven described the start of the programme as 'a light in this darkness'.[120] In early-2021, the ambition would have to be pushed back a bit.

Löfven Caught Breaking the Rules

In the dying days of 2020, Löfven had brought a spotlight down on himself when he joined a long roll-call of political leaders and policy makers around the world who had encouraged criticism over breaking coronavirus measures that they themselves had put in place or had supported. Accusations of double standards over restrictions and lockdowns were levelled.

In the UK, in spring, Dominic Cummings, the chief adviser to Boris Johnson, had faced calls to resign after driving almost the entire length of England which was against the restrictions on movement that were in place at the time. He believed himself and his family to be displaying COVID-19 symptoms, and rather than self-isolate at home – which he should have done – he had driven his wife and child north to be close to family in county Durham for help with childcare. Additionally, while there, a visit by car to Barnard Castle attracted widespread ridicule.

In March, the Spanish vice-president, Pablo Iglesias, faced public condemnation for breaking rules on self-isolation after carrying on working, despite his partner having had a positive test for coronavirus, and in quarantine. Later he had been photographed without a mask at a supermarket, which was against government guidelines.

In Poland, in April, the prime minister, Mateusz Morawiecki, joined a public gathering to remember the dead of the 2010 Smolensk air crash. He had not been wearing a mask, and the gathering was viewed as violating the lockdown.

In Ireland, in May, the prime minister Leo Varadkar had been photographed enjoying a picnic with his partner and friends in a park and had been criticised for setting a bad example. Also in May, in Austria, the president, Alexander van der Bellen, had been caught by police breaking curfew by staying late at a restaurant. Earlier, the Austrian Chancellor, Sebastian Kurz faced condemnation after a visit to a small border community attracted a crowd that flouted social distancing rules. Public gatherings of more than ten had been banned and only a handful in the crowd had worn masks.

In Germany, in May, Christian Lindner, the liberal FDP leader (the Free Democrats, Free Democratic Party), had been caught hugging a friend outside a restaurant in violation of social distancing rules.

In Scotland, in December, the first minister, Nicola Sturgeon (to all intents and purposes the Scottish prime minister), faced criticism after removing her mask during a wake to converse with other attendees after the funeral of a government civil servant. She said that regardless of the circumstances she was in the wrong, and there were no excuses.

Also in December, Löfven, together with his bodyguards, had been spotted at the 'Gallerian' shopping mall in central Stockholm just a couple of days after urging Swedes to avoid crowded places and do their part in curbing the spread of coronavirus. The prime minister had been collecting an item from a watchmaker, after earlier visits to the mall during December. At the time of these earlier visits to 'Gallerian', the local recommendations stated that people should refrain from spending time in indoor environments such as shops, shopping centres, museums, libraries, pools, and gyms. Löfven himself had made it clear that the rules were to be followed at all times. While the rules did not prohibit visits to shopping centres and malls, his critics suggested that he should be held to a higher standard. His actions undermined the entire strategy, and there was a chance that his message next time might not be taken seriously. In an article headline, the newspaper *Expressen* screamed: 'Löfven has shopped away his credibility'.[121]

Löfven had not been the only Swedish politician or public figure facing criticism. The justice minister, Morgan Johansson, had visited the 'Nova Lund' shopping centre in Lund, southern Sweden, just after Christmas, and the finance minister Magdalena Andersson, had visited the ski resort of Sälen in Region Dalarna. The head of the Civil Contingencies Agency (*Myndigheten för samhällsskydd och beredskap, MSB*), Dan Eliasson, who had been heavily involved in communication about coronavirus, was seen on a flight to the Canary Islands in mid-December. While neither Andersson's nor Eliasson's trips were illegal, non-essential travel had been discouraged, and in early-January 2021, Ulf Kristersson, leader of the Moderates and the centre-right opposition, was calling for Eliasson's resignation, describing the trip as 'an abdication of responsibility'. Eliasson was moved over to the crisis preparedness division at the justice ministry.[122]

In late-September, Ebba Busch, leader of the Christian Democrats, became the centre of discussion after being seen dancing, hugging, and kissing at a 40th birthday party, shortly after Löfven had warned of the risks that partying could bring amid rising infection rates. Jimmie Åkesson, leader of the Sweden Democrats, had also been caught out at a party – a 50th birthday party in Öxelösund – where he had been photographed throwing his arm round guests.[123] All this against the backdrop of rising coronavirus infection rates, and deaths.

Statistics, Year End 2020

Since the start of the coronavirus outbreak, cumulative deaths across the Nordic countries by end-December had been recorded as: in Sweden 8,727, Denmark 1,298, Finland 561, Norway 436, and in Iceland 29.

While Sweden's figures had been clearly very much worse than its close neighbours, in comparison to those recorded in Hungary and Czechia, one slightly smaller in population (Hungary) and the other (Czechia) slightly larger, they stood up well. Hungary had recorded 9,537 deaths, and Czechia 11,580. Relative to population at end-December, Sweden's recorded deaths had been 858.94 per million, whereas Hungary had recorded 989.91, and Czechia 1,079.77.

At the start of the pandemic, the country's maverick approach was losing it many lives to the virus and causing it to stand out as the 'outlier', but by the end of 2020, recorded deaths to COVID-19 were starting to 'look normal' when compared with countries outside the Nordic region.[124]

In the rest of Europe, Italy, the UK, France, Russia, and Spain had recorded the highest number of cumulative deaths by end-December, each country recording between 50,000 and 75,000 victims. In Italy the figure was 74,159, and in the UK 73,570, the milestone of 70,000 UK deaths having been passed 24–25 December. In France the number of deaths had been 64,644, in Russia 56,271 and in Spain 50,837. In the UK, the 75,000 milestone was passed 2–3 January 2021. In China, where the virus had been first identified, there had been only 4,634 deaths claimed since January 2020.[125]

Cumulatively worldwide, some 1.88 million people had died from COVID-19 since January 2020. In the continent of Europe, there had been 545,520 deaths over 2020, and in the EU, 370,470. In North America there had been 512,711 deaths, in South America 418,041, in Asia 337,854, in Africa 65,468, and in Australia 909.[126]

Chapter 6 will take a brief step backwards to consider not only how the maverick Swedish approach to COVID-19 became a symbol in national debates elsewhere, but how throughout the twentieth century and into the twenty-first century the Swedish approach to many things had been held up in political discourse as an example that should not be followed. It examines how the creation of a negative image of Sweden had long served as a political tool in democracies around the world. Just what was it about Sweden? Why was 'Sweden-bashing' the often-used tool of politicians on the American right?

Notes

1 'Statement on the fourth meeting of the International Health Regulations (2005) Emergency Committee regarding the outbreak of coronavirus disease (COVID-19)', World Health Organization (WHO), 1 August 2020, <https://www.who.int/news/-room/detail/01-08-2020-statement-on-the-fourth-meeting-of-the-international-health-regulations-(2005)-emergency-committee-regarding-the-outbreak-of-coronavirus-disease-(covid-19)> accessed 3 August 2020, and, Baynes, Chris. 'Coronavirus pandemic will be lengthy, World Health Organisation warns', *The Independent*, 2 August 2020, <https://www.independent.co.uk/news/world/coronavirus-pandemic-lengthy-world-health-organisation-emergency-committee-a9649841.html> accessed 3 August 2020.

2 Henley, Jon. 'Global report: France could lose control of Covid-19 at any time', *The Guardian*, 4 August 2020, <http://www.theguardian.com/world/2020/aug/04/global-report-france-could-lose-control-of-covid-19-at-any-time> accessed 6 August 2020.

3 'Cumulative confirmed COVID-19 cases' & 'Cumulative confirmed COVID-19 deaths', August 1, 2020', Our World in Data, COVID-19 dataset, <https://ourworldindata.org> accessed 15 December 2021.

4 ‘Daily new confirmed COVID-19 cases per million people, August 1, 2020’, Our World in Data, COVID-19 dataset, <http://ourworldindata.org> accessed 15 December 2021.

5 Ibid.

6 ‘Cumulative confirmed COVID-19 deaths, August 31, 2020’, Our World in Data, COVID-19 dataset, <https://ourworldindata.org> accessed 15 December 2021.

7 ‘Covid-19 news: Europe faces tricky moment as coronavirus cases climb’, *New Scientist*, 27 August 2020, <https://www.newscientist.com/article/2237475-covid-19-news-europe-faces-tricky-moment-as-coronavirus-cases-climb/> accessed 28 August 2020.

8 ‘Cumulative confirmed COVID-19 cases, August 31, 2020’, Our World in Data, COVID-19 dataset, <https://ourworldindata.org> accessed 15 December 2021.

9 ‘Coronavirus: WHO warns Europe over very serious Covid surge’, *BBC News*, 18 September 2020, < https://www.bbc.co.uk/news/world-europe-54 189575> accessed 19 September 2020.

10 ‘Cumulative confirmed COVID-19 cases, September 19, 2020’, and ‘Cumulative confirmed COVID-19 deaths, September 30, 2020’, Our World in Data, COVID-19 dataset <https://ourworldindata.org> accessed 15 December 2021.

11 ‘Daily new confirmed COVID-19 cases per million people, September 30, 2020’, Our World in Data, COVID-19 dataset <https://ourworldindata.org> accessed 16 December 2021.

12 ‘Cumulative confirmed COVID-19 deaths, September 30, 2020’, Our World in Data, COVID-19 dataset <https://ourworldindata.org> accessed 16 December 2021.

13 Woolhouse, Mark. ‘We should follow the Swedes and learn to live with the virus’, *Telegraph*, Sunday 20 September 2020, p. 5.

14 Ibid.

15 Ibid.

16 Ibid.

17 ‘Folkhälsomyndigheten har misslyckats – nu måste politkerna gripa in’, *Dagens Nyheter*, 14 April 2020, <https://www.dn.se/debatt/folkhalsomyndigheten-har-misslyckats-nu-maste-politikerna-gripa-in/> accessed 24 April 2020.

18 Vogel, Gretchen. ‘It’s been so, so surreal. Critics of Sweden’s lax pandemic policies face fierce backlash’, *Science*, AAAS.org (American Association for the Advancement of Science), 6 October 2020, <https://www.sciencemag.org/news/2020/10/it-s-been-so-so-surreal-critics-sweden-s-lax-pandemic-policies-face-fierce-backlash> accessed 24 November 2020.

19 ‘COVID-19 in Europe. A patchwork of red, yellow and green’, *The Economist*, 24–30 October 2020, Vol. 437, No. 9217, p. 31.

20 Looi, Mun-Keat. ‘Covid-19: Is a second wave hitting Europe?’ *British Medical Journal, BMJ*, 28 October 2020, <https://www.bmj.com/content/371/bmj.m4113> accessed 9 November 2020.

21 *The Economist*, 24–30 October 2020, as note 19, p. 32.

22 Looi, as note 20.

23 ‘Cumulative confirmed COVID-19 cases, October 21, 2020’, Our World in Data, COVID-19 dataset<https://ourworldindata.org> accessed 16 December 2021.

24 Looi, as note 20.

25 ‘Questions & answers on the coordination of measures restricting free movement in the European Union related to the coronavirus pandemic’, Press corner, European Commission, 13 October 2020, <https://ec.europa.eu/commission/presscorner/detail/en/QANDA_20_1875> accessed 28 October 2020.

26 Ibid.

[27] *The Economist*, 24–30 October 2020, as note 19, p. 32.

[28] 'Combined indicator: 14-day notification rate, testing rate and test positivity, updated 22 October 2020', <https://www.ecdc.europa.eu/en/covid-19/situation-updates/weekly-maps-coordinated-restriction-free-movement> accessed 29 October 2020.

[29] Ibid.

[30] Ibid.

[31] Ibid.

[32] '14-day case notification rate per 100,000 inhabitants, updated 22 October 2020', <https://www.ecdc.europa.eu/covid-19/situation-updates/weekly-maps-coordinated-restriction-free-movement> accessed 27 October 2020.

[33] Ibid.

[34] Ibid.

[35] 'Covid: Merkel warns of long hard winter as lockdowns return', *BBC News*, 29 October 2020, <https://www.bbc.co.uk/news/world-europe-54728893> accessed 30 October.

[36] 'EU to fund transfer of COVID-19 patients across borders to prevent hospitals collapse', *Reuters*, 29 October 2020, <https://uk.reuters.com/article/uk-health-coronavirus-eu-overwhelmed/eu-at-risk-of-being-overwhelmed-by-coronavirus-eu-commission-head-idUKKBN27E3JZ> accessed 30 October 2020.

[37] 'Sweden's coronavirus measures could remain in place for at least another year', *The Local*, 5 October 2020, <https://www.thelocal.se/20201005/swedens-coronavirus-measures-could-remain-in-place-for-at-least-another-year> accessed 30 October 2020.

[38] Woodcock, Andrew. 'Coronavirus: Second wave could last until April in worst case scenario, leaked document reveals', *Independent*, 29 October 2020, <https://www.independent.co.uk/news/uk/politics-/coronavirus-second-wave-worst-case-sage-boris-johnson-lockdown-b140378.html> accessed 30 October 2020.

[39] 'Combined indicator: 14-day notification rate, testing rate and test positivity, updated 19 November 2020', <https://www.ecdc.europa.eu/en/covid-19/situation-updates/weekly-maps-coordinated-restriction-free-movement> accessed 24 November 2020.

[40] Edwards, Catherine. 'Is it right to say Sweden is still not experiencing a second wave of COVID-19', *The Local*, 16 October 2020, <https://www.thelocal.se/20201016/is-it-right-to-say-sweden-is-still-not-experiencing-a-second-wave-of-the-coronavirus> accessed 30 October 2020.

[41] Ibid.

[42] Ibid.

[43] 'Get a grip! Swedish minister tells students off after university outbreaks', *The Local*, 9 October 2020, <https://www.thelocal.se/20201009/get-a-grip-swedish-minister-tells-students-off-after-university-outbreaks> accessed 30 October 2020.

[44] 'Sweden and Covid-19. Land of the mask-free', p. 14. & 'Coronavirus in Sweden. The odd one out', *The Economist*, 10–16 October 2020, Vol. 437, No. 9215, p. 34.

[45] 'Sweden and Covid-19. Land of the mask-free', p. 14, and 'Coronavirus in Sweden. The odd one out', p. 34, *The Economist*, 10–16 October 2020.

[46] Norberg, Johan. 'Sweden during the pandemic. Pariah or paragon?' p. 10, *CATO policy analysis*, No. 959, 29 August 2023, Cato Institute, <https://www.cato.org/sites/cato.org/files/2023-08/policy-analysis-959-no-link.pdf> accessed 6 February 2025.

[47] Ibid.

[48] Löfgren, Emma. 'New coronavirus measures rolled out in three Swedish regions, including Stockholm and Gothenburg', *The Local*, 29 October 2020, <https://www.thelocal.se/20201029/new-coronavirus-measures-for-three-swedish-regions-including-stockholm-and-gothenburg> accessed 29 October 2020.

49 'Coronavirus: The latest news about the outbreak in Sweden', *The Local*, updated 29 October 2020, <https://www.thelocal.se/20200902/coronavirus-the-latest-news-about-the-outbreak-in-sweden-timeline-part-two> accessed 29 October 2020.

50 Ibid.

51 Eaton, George. 'Trust is vital if you want to stop this disease', Anders Tegnell on leading Sweden's fight against Covid-19, p. 17, *New Statesman*, 23–29 October 2020, p. 16–17.

52 Edwards, Catherine. 'Analysis: Is Sweden heading for a national lockdown?', *The Local*, 6 November 2020, <https://www.thelocal.se/20201106/is-sweden-heading-for-a-national-lockdown> accessed 7 November 2020.

53 Ewald, Hugo. and Hans Olsson, 'Stefan Löven i karantän', *Dagens Nyheter*, 6 November 2020, <https://www.dn.se/sverige/stefan-lofven-i-karantan/> accessed 16 December 2021.

54 Ibid.

55 Lagerwall, Katarina. 'Fler minkbesättningar i Sverige smittade av coronavirus', *Dagens Nyheter*, 5 November 2020, <https://www.dn.se/sverige/fler-minkbesattningar-i-sverige-smittade-av-coronavirus/> and, 'Denmark to cull up to 17 million mink amid coronavirus fears', *BBC News*, 5 November 2020, <https://www.bbc.co.uk/news/world-europe-54818615> accessed 6 November 2020.

56 'Coronavirus: Denmark imposes lockdowns amid mink covid fears', *BBC News*, 6 November 2020, <https://www.bbc.co.uk/news/world-europe-54833459> accessed 7 November 2020.

57 Lagerwall, as note 55.

58 Ibid.

59 *BBC News*, 6 November 2020, as note 56.

60 Lawton, Graham. 'Is a dangerous new coronavirus strain circulating in farmed mink?' *New Scientist*, 6 November 2020, <https://www.newscientist.com/article/2259178-is-a-dangerous-new-coronavirus-strain-circulating-in-farmed-mink/> accessed 7 November 2020.

61 James, Liam. 'What is mink-related coronavirus?' *Independent*, 7 November 2020, <https://www.independent.co.uk/news/world/europe/coronavirus-mink-denmark-cull-vaccine-b1641128.html> accessed 9 November 2020.

62 Mallapaty, Smriti. 'Covid mink analysis shows mutations are not dangerous – yet', *Nature*, No. 587, pp. 340–41, 13 November 2020), <https://doi.org/10.1038/d41586-020-03218-z> accessed 14 December 2020.

63 Henley, Jon. 'Decomposing mink in Denmark may have contaminated groundwater', *The Guardian*, 10 December 2020, <https://www.theguardian.com/world/2020/dec/10/decomposing-mink-in-denmark-may-have-contaminated-groundwater> accessed 10 December 2020.

64 'Sweden halts mink breeding over coronavirus concerns', *The Local*, 27 January 2021, <https://www.thelocal.se/20210127/sweden-halts-mink-breeding-over-coronavirus-concerns> accessed 28 January 2021.

65 'Cumulative confirmed COVID-19 cases, October 31, 2020', and 'Cumulative confirmed COVID-19 deaths, October 31, 2020', Our World in Data, COVID-19 dataset, <https://ourworldindata.org> accessed 16 December 2021.

66 'Cumulative confirmed COVID-19 deaths, October 31, 2020', Our World in Data, COVID-19 dataset, <https://ourworldindata.org> accessed 16 December 2021.

67 Ibid.

68 'Daily new confirmed COVID-19 deaths per million people, October 31, 2020', Our World in Data, COVID-19 dataset, <https://ourworldindata.org> accessed 16 December 2021.

69 ‘Daily new confirmed COVID-19 cases per million people, October 31, 2020’, Our World in Data, COVID-19 dataset, <https://ourworldindata.org> accessed 16 December 2021.

70 ‘Covid: UK first country in Europe to pass 50,000 deaths’, *BBC News*, 11 November 2020, <https://www.bbc.co.uk/news/uk-54905018> and, ‘Cumulative confirmed COVID-19 deaths per million people, November 11, 2020’, Our World in Data, COVID-19 dataset, <https://ourworldindata.org> accessed 16 December 2021.

71 ‘Cumulative confirmed COVID-19 deaths per million people, November 19, 2020’, Our World in Data, COVID-19 dataset, <https://ourworldindata.org> accessed 16 December 2021.

72 ‘More Swedish regions introduce stricter coronavirus measures’, *The Local*, 10 November 2020, <https://www.thelocal.se/20201110/more-regions-introduce-local-coronavirus-recommendations> accessed 28 November 2020.

73 ‘Sweden to ban sale of alcohol after 10pm’, *The Local*, 11 November 2020, <https://www.thelocal.se/20201111/breaking-sweden-to-ban-sale-of-alcohol-after-10pm> accessed 28 November 2020.

74 ‘EU could see Covid-19 vaccinations rolled out first quarter next year’, *The Local*, 11 November 2020, <https://www.thelocal.se/20201111/eu-could-see-first-covid-19-vaccinations-first-quarter-next-year> accessed 28 November 2020.

75 ‘Explained: What does Sweden’s new limit on public events actually mean?’ *The Local*, 16 November 2020, <https://www.thelocal.se/20201116/explained-what-does-swedens-new-limit-on-public-events-actually-mean> accessed 29 November 2020.

76 ‘Stockholm and Malmö shut gyms, museums and swimming pools’, *The Local*, 20 November 2020, <https://www.thelocal.se/20201120/stockholm-and-malmo-shut-gyms-museums-and-swimming-pools> accessed 29 November 2020.

77 ‘WHO: Countries like Sweden should consider face masks’, *The Local*, 17 November 2020, <https://www.thelocal.se/20201117/world-health-organisation-urges-like-sweden-should-consider-face-masks> accessed 29 November 2020.

78 ‘Ny rapport om munskydd och ventilation från Vetenskapsakademiens expertgrupp om Covid-19’, Press release, Kungl. Vetenskapsakademien, 19 November 2020, <https://www.kva.se/sv/pressrum/pressmedelanden/ny-rapport-om-munskydd-och-ventilation-fran-vetenskapsakademiens-expertgrupp-om-covid-19> accessed 29 November 2020.

79 ‘Prime Minister Stefan Löfven’s address to the nation’ / ‘Statsminister Stefan Löfvens tal till nationen’, Government Offices of Sweden, Stockholm, 22 November 2020, <https://www.government.se/speeches/2020/11/prime-minister-stefan-lofvens-address-to-the-nation- sunday-22-november/> accessed 29 November 2020.

80 Ibid.

81 Ibid.

82 Ibid.

83 ‘Swedish royals test positive for Covid-19’, *The Local*, 26 November 2020, <https://www.thelocal.se/20201126/swedish-royals-test-positive-for-covid-19> accessed 10 December 2020.

84 Habib, Heba. ‘COVID-19: What Sweden taught Scandinavia for the second wave’, *British Medical Journal*, *BMJ*, 27 November 2020, <https://doi.org/10.1136/bmj.m4456> accessed 30 November 2020.

85 Ibid.

86 Ibid.

87 Ibid.

88 Ibid.

89 'New scenario: Sweden's coronavirus outbreak may peak in December', *The Local*, 26 November 2020, <https://www.thelocal.se/20201126/new-scenario-swedens-coronavirus-outbreak-may-peak-in-december> accessed 10 December 2020.

90 Ibid., and, 'Cumulative confirmed COVID-19 deaths, November 30, 2020', Our World in Data, COVID-19 dataset, <https://ourworldindata.org> accessed 16 December 2021.

91 'Sverige har återigen överdödlighet – äldre hårdast drabbade', Press release, SCB, 14 December 2020, <https://www.scb.se/om-scb/nyheter-och-pressmeddelanden/sverige-har-aterigen-overdodlighet--aldre-hardast-drabbade> and, 'Sweden records deadliest November in a century', *The Local*, 14 December 2020, <https://www.thelocal.se/20201214/sweden-sees-highest-excess-mortality-in-100-years> accessed 27 December 2020.

92 'Cumulative confirmed COVID-19 deaths, November 30, 2020', Our World in Data, COVID-19 dataset, <https://ourworldindata.org> accessed 16 December 2021.

93 'Daily new confirmed COVID-19 deaths per million people, November 30, 2020', Our World in Data, COVID-19 dataset, <https://ourworldindata.org> accessed 16 December 2021.

94 'Daily new confirmed COVID-19 cases per million people, November 30, 2020', Our World in Data, COVID-19 dataset, <https://ourworldindata.org> accessed 16 December 2021.

95 'Cumulative confirmed COVID-19 deaths per million people', December 3, 2020, Our World in Data, COVID-19 dataset, <https://ourworldindata.org> accessed 16 December 2021.

96 'Covax: Working for global equitable access to COVID-19 vaccines', World Health Organization, <https://www.who.int/initiatives/act-accelerator/covax> and, 'UN welcomes nearly $1 billion in recent pledges – to bolster access to lifesaving tests, treatments and vaccines to end Covid-19', UN Office for the Coordination of Humanitarian Affairs (OCHA), reliefweb, 30 September 2020, <https://reliefweb.int/report/world/un-welcomes-nearly-1-billion-recent-pledges-bolster-access-lifesaving-tests-treatments> accessed 15 December 2020.

97 'Overview of Covid-19 vaccination strategies and vaccine deployment in the EU/EEA and the UK', Technical report, European Centre for Disease Prevention and Control (ECDC), 2 December 2020, p. 7, and p. 11, <https://www.ecdc.europa.eu/sites/default/files/documents/Overview-of-EU_EEA-UK-vaccination-deployment-plans.pdf> accessed 8 December 2020.

98 Ibid., p. 13, and p. 23.

99 'FAQ about COVID-19', Folkhälsomyndigheten / Public Health Agency of Sweden, 8 December 2020, <https://www.folkhalsomyndigheten.se/the-public-health-agency-of-sweden/communicable-disease-control/covid-19/covid-19-faq/> accessed 8 December 2020.

100 'First batch of COVID-19 vaccine now to arrive in Sweden by Christmas', *Sveriges Radio* / Radio Sweden, 16 December 2020, <https://sverigesradio.se/artikel/7626291> accessed 27 December 2020.

101 'COVID: Are countries under pressure to approve vaccine?', *BBC News*, 3 December 2020, <https://www.bbc.co.uk/news/world-55175232> accessed 27 December 2020. The woman who was the first person in the world to receive the coronavirus vaccine was Margaret Keenan, given it at the Coventry university hospital (University Hospital Coventry and Warwickshire) when she was 90. By the time she got the follow-up second dose three weeks later she had become 91-years old.

102 Murphy, Flynn. 'Inside China's response to Covid', *Nature*, 2 December 2020, No. 588, pp. 49–51, <https://doi.org/10.1038/d41586-020-03361-7> accessed 19 December 2020.

103 'For the first time since spring, more than half of Sweden's ICU patients have Covid- 19', *The Local*, 1 December 2020, <https://ww.thelocal.se/20201201/for-the-first-time-since-spring-more-than-half-of-swedens-icu-patients-have-covid-19> accessed 11 December 2020.

104 'Stockholm healthcare chief calls for help from public as ICUs reach 99 percent capacity', *The Local*, 9 December 2020, <https://www.thelocal.se/20201209/stockholms-icu-units-reach-99-percent-capacity/> accessed 11 December 2020.

105 'Is the second wave overloading Sweden's intensive care units?' *The Local*, 11 December 2020, <http://www.thelocal.se/20201211/is-the-second-wave-overloading-swedens-intensive-care-units> accessed 12 December 2020.

106 'Sweden's schools for over-16s shift back to remote learning', *The Local*, 3 December 2020, <https://www.thelocal.se/20201203/swedens-schools-for-over16s-shift-back-to-remote-learning> accessed 11 December 2020.

107 Ibid.

108 'Stockholm shuts schools for 13- to 15-year-olds for first time due to coronavirus', *The Local*, 11 December 2020, <https://www.thelocal.se/20201211/stockholm-shuts-schools-to-13-to-15-year-old-for-first-time> accessed 12 December 2020.

109 'Stay in your bubble: Swedish leaders warn of Christmas coronavirus peak', *The Local*, 8 December 2020, <https://www.thelocal.se/20201208/stay-in-your-bubble-swedish-leaders-warn-of-christmas-coronavirus-peak> accessed 11 December 2020.

110 Ibid.

111 Ibid.

112 Löfgren, Emma. 'Sweden rolls out series of new coronavirus measures, including face masks', *The Local*, 18 December 2020, <https://www.thelocal.se/20201218/swedish-prime-minister-stefan-lofven-press-conference-coronavirus> accessed 27 December 2020.

113 'Explained: When and where do you need to wear a face mask in Sweden?', *The Local*, 30 December 2020, <https://www.thelocal.se/20201230/this-is-swedens-new-face-mask-recommendation> accessed 30 December 2020.

114 'Covid: WHO in close contact with UK over new virus variant', *BBC News*, 21 December 2020, <https://www.bbc.co.uk/news/world-55382212> accessed 27 December 2020.

115 Ibid.

116 'Coronavirus: Cases of new variant appear worldwide', *BBC News*, 27 December 2020, <https://www.bbc.co.uk/news/world-europe-55452262> accessed 27 December 2020.

117 'Covid: Pfizer-BioNTech vaccine approved for EU states', *BBC News*, 22 December 2020, <https://www.bbc.co.uk/news/world-europe-55401136> accessed 27 December 2020.

118 'Covid: EU starts mass vaccination in touching moment of unity', *BBC News*, 27 December 2020, <https://www.bbc.co.uk/news/world-europe-55456795> accessed 27 December 2020.

119 'Czech PM receives vaccine as EU roll-out gets under way', *RTÉ News*, 27 December 2020, <https://www.rte.ie/news/world/2020/1227/1186587-europe-covid-vaccine/> accessed 28 December 2020.

120 Emanuelsson, Eric, and Stjernberg, Max Sohl. 'Gun-Britt Johnsson, 91, först i Sverige med att få vaccin', *Expressen*, 27 December 2020, <https://www.expressen.se/nyheter/coronaviruset/har-far-gun-britt-91-vaccinet-mot-corona1/> accessed 28 December 2020.

121 Holm, Gusten. Stjernberg, Max Stohl. and Ingmo, Daniel. 'Bilderna avslöjar: Här julbesöker Löfven Gallerian', *Expressen*, 29 December 2020, <https://www.expressen.se/nyheter/coronaviruset/bilderna-avslojar-har-julbesoker-lofven-gallerian> and, 'Löfven har shoppat bort sin trovärdighet', *Expressen*, editorial, 29 December 2020, <https://www.expressen.se/ledare/lofven-har-shoppat-bort-sin-trovardighet/> accessed 30 December 2020.

[122] 'Swedish party head calls for crisis chief to resign over Canaries trip', *The Local*, 6 January 2021, <https://www.thelocal.se/20210106/swedish-opposition-calls-for-crisis-chief-to-resign-over-christmas-trip> accessed 6 January 2021.

[123] 'Swedish Prime Minister Stefan Löfven criticised over pre-Christmas shopping centre visit', *The Local*, 29 December 2020, <https://www.thelocal.se/20201229/swedish-prime-minister-stafanlfven-faces-criticism-over-pre-christmas-shopping-centre-visit> accessed 30 December 2020.

[124] 'Cumulative confirmed COVID-19 deaths, December 31, 2020', and 'Cumulative confirmed COVID-19 deaths per million people, December 31 2020', Our World in Data, COVID-19 dataset, <https://ourworldindata.org> accessed 17 December 2021.

[125] Ibid.

[126] Ibid.

Sweden the Maverick? Sweden a Cautionary Tale?

Sweden 2020

Quiet streets but not deserted. Outdoor cafes open, the young socializing closely in parks. This had been Sweden in the spring of the first year of the COVID-19 pandemic – 2020.

While Stefan Löfven had talked of tough weeks and months ahead in his address to the nation in March 2020, Swedes were being allowed a fair degree of personal freedom and not being locked down at home. While on the one hand social distancing and working from home had been advised, on the other, restaurants and bars could remain open and serve people at tables. For older students, upper schools, colleges, and universities had been closed, but for younger students and infants, primary school classes and nurseries remained open.

Some had asserted that Sweden's approach had been informed by science, and that the actions of other countries were ill-judged, unconsidered – groping in the dark – and based on politics. Nevertheless, Sweden did certainly seem to be the 'outlier', the 'outrider', the 'maverick', especially when judged against death rates and case numbers in Nordic and Baltic neighbours.

While Löfven and the government trusted the population to act responsibly, scientists had criticised the strategy of the public health agency as irresponsible. In response, the agency had argued that if the country's approach seemed anomalous, it was more sustainable and effective in protecting the health of the public (especially mental health) than firm lockdown and closure. The goal had been to slow down the rate of infection so that healthcare and intensive care units did not become overwhelmed, and that had been the goal across Europe, though different countries chose different means to achieve that.

The Swedish 'common sense' approach which had relied on high levels of public trust in the authorities and of compliance, had drawn on the tradition of collective action in defence of Sweden and from outside threats to the country, as experienced during the Second World War.[1] The UK had not been the only country able to draw on wartime experience.

Even so, protection of the elderly and vulnerable, a core component of the Swedish strategy, had singularly failed. By autumn 2020 it was clear that nearly half of Sweden's COVID-19 deaths had taken place in care homes for the elderly.[2]

If the strategy had been pursued for economic reasons – the government had argued that it had not been – then this had failed, for the impact of the pandemic was expected to cause contraction in the economy comparable to neighbouring states.[3]

No matter the reasons behind it, the Swedish strategy towards the COVID-19 pandemic had been the subject of intense international fascination. At times the approach had been described as bold and brave, at times infamous and enlightened, at times risky and foolhardy, and Sweden was seen as a country dogged by moral superiority, making it slow to react. However, it was certainly not the first time that Sweden, or a Swedish approach, had been raised in foreign debate as an example to be avoided.

What Was it About Sweden?

The Swedish approach to tackling COVID-19 had provided endless fascination across the world. In the face of lockdown restrictions in country after country – restrictions not seen or experienced outside wartime – it had seemed that journalists only wanted to write about Sweden.[4]

The attention and scrutiny given to the country was wide-ranging, and much focus and much media copy had been given to the distinct position taken by Sweden – a dissenting approach – from its European neighbours. Serving as an exemplar was the piece by Richard Milne (*Financial Times*, 16 October 2020). Quoting Nicholas Aylott, a political scientist at Södertörn University (*Södertörns högskola*) in Huddinge, Stockholm, Milne observed that the solo approach taken by Sweden towards COVID-19 – marked by its avoidance of formal lockdown – was not dissimilar to the approach taken towards the 2015 migration crisis when it accepted more asylum seekers than any other EU member state. It seemed striking to Aylott that in only a short span of years Sweden had taken a very different approach from other countries towards two separate international crises. It had been 'a case of true Swedish exceptionalism', he posited.[5]

According to experts, at the heart of this 'outlier' stance was Sweden's sense of itself as a 'moral superpower', despite its size. Then, clearly blind to Sweden's membership of the EU for a quarter of a century – an economic and trading alliance – and its repeated foreign and security policy statements on defence solidarity with Nordic and Baltic neighbours and other members of the EU, the experts decided that 'neutrality' lay behind Sweden's stance and sense of itself. Sweden's moral superiority lay 'deeply rooted' in its 'long-held neutrality', Milne postulated. It had not fought a war for more than two centuries, leading it to 'being slow to react'.[6] It was as if neither the speech made by Carl Bildt in Bonn nearly thirty years before – effectively consigning the 'policy neutrality' to history in an address to the Office of the Commission of the European Communities in 1991 – nor three decades of carefully cultured post-neutrality after that speech had ever occurred. And besides – and there is always room for a bit of 'whataboutery' – what about the reaction time of the UK, a country constantly on the back foot in the fight against COVID-19?

Some of the fascination with Sweden lay in how it had come to symbolize the debate around 'community immunity', or 'population immunity' (more acceptable phraseology than 'herd immunity' which was loaded with negativity). As described earlier, other countries had briefly considered allowing the virus to propagate through the population in a controlled manner – the UK and the Netherlands had – but caved in to scientific and public pressure as death tolls climbed. Herd immunity had not been the goal in Sweden either, Tegnell would have been quick to point out. The overall objective had been to reduce the pace of spread of the virus so that the elderly and vulnerable could be sheltered and healthcare had a reasonable workload,[7] but this would also bring a natural immunity among the population.

'Flattening the curve' in this way had been the same strategy as taken by most other countries. However, much of Sweden's implementation had focussed on voluntary actions of a population trusting of its government, of agencies, and of authorities. Sweden had acted by degrees and given advice and recommendation rather than enacting legislation and compulsory measures, and it had been this that had drawn considerable attention in foreign media.[8]

For a time, the Swedish approach – its 'experiment' – had been hailed as bold and brave but nonetheless not without risk.[9] Several principal stories emerged in foreign writing about Sweden. Sometimes it was a case of life being 'normal' with the story accompanied by images of people socializing in street cafes and going about their daily business or showing schools open and people strolling about in spring sunshine, and sometimes it was about Sweden's herd immunity strategy. Sometimes the story was about how Sweden was not following expert advice and not following WHO recommendations. Sometimes the story was about the failure of the Swedish approach, and sometimes it was about the trust Swedes had in their governments.[10]

Surely though, Tegnell and Carlson were experts in their field too – one was the chief epidemiologist, the other the director-general of the public health agency. What had guided them in their decision-making was in-depth and expert knowledge, said Carlson. They set about their work based on science and evidence.

That Sweden had been written about as the 'outlier' by foreign journalists, both frightened and fascinated him in good measure, but he could understand why it aroused curiosity. However, he believed that 'Sweden the outlier' was a myth. Things had not been done that differently in Sweden. What had made the difference was rhetoric and language. Of course, there were countries which had done drastically different things, with draconian bans, but the approach Sweden had taken was less lax than described by journalists. It was important that any measures put in place had the acceptance of the population, otherwise compliance would be hard to achieve, he said. Politicians had to understand that. He acknowledged and pointed to the fact that there had been some ambivalence towards Sweden's way of handling the pandemic. Sometimes it had been viewed as exciting to learn from and sometimes seen as a threat because it could directly undermine some drastic measures taken in their own countries.[11]

Mounting death statistics into March 2020 ensured the hegemony of lockdown strategies, ending the 'lockdown' versus 'herd immunity' debate, and by June the media – and indeed politicians – would be 'interpreting and conveying a negative moral judgement' on the Swedish strategy. In the end, Sweden would achieve pariah status – no longer bold and brave.[12]

While there had been a fascination for Sweden and its strategy towards COVID-19, role model it was not. When asked in a daily press conference about following the Swedish method of handling the pandemic and its model of looser restrictions than in other countries (reported on 11 April 2020), the American president, Donald Trump, had been quick to downplay any benefits of doing so, and condemned Sweden's approach. Sweden was 'suffering very greatly', he said. Sweden was 'suffering very very badly' (Trump never offered statesman-like rhetoric). While some conservative writers in the USA had pointed to Sweden as a champion of maintaining some economic activity during the crisis, Trump held up Sweden as an example of what countries should not be doing.[13]

But it had not been the first time that Sweden had been used in this fashion; it had not been the first time that Sweden or a 'Swedish approach' had been held up in national debates as an example that should not be followed. Creating a negative image of Sweden – 'Sweden-bashing' – had long served as a useful tool in political discourse around the world and had been so from the first Trump presidency and right back to the Johnson and Nixon presidencies at the height of the Vietnam War in the late-1960s, and to Eisenhower in the 1950s, and then forward again to Viktor Orbán and Jarosław Kaczyński in Hungary and Poland more recently. The issues raised had been as diverse as, in our own contemporary period, Sweden's approach to COVID-19, migration, rapes, Sharia law and no-go areas, and during earlier post-war years, morality, neutrality, suicide, drunkenness, the welfare state, high taxation, and state bureaucracy.

No, you did not want to be like Sweden.

Donald Trump on Sweden – Migrants

During a political campaign rally in Melbourne, Florida on 18 February 2017, and concerning the wider debate on immigration to the USA and the related discussion over the terror threat facing Europe after large-scale immigration, Trump had set off varying degrees of confusion and controversy after referring to 'what's happening last night in Sweden'. Who would have believed this of Sweden? he asked, referring to migrants. 'They took in large numbers. They're having problems like they never thought possible', he went on.[14]

His confusing comments brought ridicule and mockery because there had been neither security incidents nor terror incidents in Sweden on the 'last night' in question – 17 February 2017. After the backlash, the President explained that he had been referring to a Friday night Fox News broadcast on Swedish immigration, refugees, and crime generally, and so not to a particular incident happening 'last night'. A White House spokesperson explained that the President had been talking about rising crime and recent incidents and had not meant to say 'last night'.[15]

In Sweden itself, Carl Bildt had queried what the President might have 'been smoking' prior to his comment. For her part Margot Wallström – foreign minister at the time – referred to how increased 'false information' about Sweden was the unfortunate and 'general tendency'. The Swedish foreign service and its embassies were 'working continuously to spread an accurate and fair picture of Sweden'.[16]

During his speech at the Florida rally, Trump announced that he would take further measures to prevent Muslims from visiting the USA. In the promotion of these restrictive policies, he had chosen to paint a dark picture of Sweden: 'look what's happening last night in Sweden'. But then, Donald Trump had not been the first foreign leader to spread false rumours about Sweden.[17]

His throwaway comment had been a failed attempt at deflection technique.

Creating a Negative Image of Sweden – Morality

It was no coincidence that Sweden had been targeted and held up as an example by the Trump administration to make the case for a crackdown on migration.

Historically, for many American Republicans, Sweden was the symbol of everything that was wrong with Europe: its openness to refugees, feminism, environmental conscience, and resistance to the Vietnam War in the 1970s.[18]

For Trump too, the progressive government of Sweden probably represented everything that he disliked: feminism, big government, multilateralism, and environmentalism.[19]

'Sweden-bashing' was an often-used tool of politicians on the American right. Creating a negative image of Sweden in the twenty-first century played into a long tradition of criticism from conservative America. Negativity was in circulation during the early years of the Cold War when American journalist Joe David Brown (1915–76) described 'Swedish sin' in his article in *Time* in 1955.[20] False reporting on high Swedish alcoholism, suicide rate, and divorce rate further fed the negative moral picture of Sweden.[21]

On sexuality morality, critics in the 1950s would point to the widely distributed Swedish films featuring nudity and implied sex scenes.[22] Together with the early filmography of Ingmar Bergman (1918–2007), Sweden rapidly earned the reputation as a country 'with malleable standards of morality'. Then, played out during that decade, the very public affair between Ingrid Bergman (1915–82) and Italian film director Roberto Rossellini (1906–77), and her battle for a divorce from her husband in Sweden – neurosurgeon Petter Lindström (1907–2000) – and then the battle for contact with her young daughter Pia Lindström (who as an adult became a television broadcaster), whipped America into a moralistic frenzy,[23] and offered another suitable setting for negativity.

Into the 1960s, Sweden's image would be coloured further by Bergman's work featuring, for the time, controversial sex scenes. Also, by the work of Vilgot Sjöman (1924–2006), dealing with class, morality, and sexual taboos, and that of Luigi Scattini (1927–2010).[24]

Then of course, there was the matter of that other dirty word, the 'n-word', that of Sweden's neutrality, and its spurning of NATO membership – not the moral choice in the view of conservative America during the Cold War. Neutrality represented deviance, escapism, and weakness; it was a policy that signalled indecisiveness. Neutrality was to be regarded as absolutely nothing to be copied.

Dwight D. Eisenhower on Sweden – Governmental Paternalism

The 'Sweden-bashing' tool was used by Dwight D. Eisenhower (1890–1969) towards the end of his Republican presidency when he tried to use his broad base of popularity to boost the presidential campaign of his vice-president, Richard Nixon (1913–94).

The Democratic opponent at the time was the formidable John F. Kennedy (1917–63) who had already knocked out Hubert Humphrey (1911–78) and other contenders. In July 1960, in a speech to delegates during the party convention in Chicago, Eisenhower had referred to the unprecedented prosperity of the USA and to how there were more Americans in work and earning higher wages than ever before in history – though he ignored the intense stratification of American society and the plight of Black and Hispanic Americans. The fruits of this success, he believed, had lain in *laissez-faire* capitalism, and not in any liberal, free-spending, governmental stimulation of the economy. Later, speaking to hundreds of selected Republicans in Chicago, and illustrating the dangers of social and political liberalism, he referred to 'a fairly friendly European country' about which he had been reading – the country was Sweden – and how its 'experiment of almost complete paternalism' had resulted in a huge rate of suicide and twice as much drunkenness than in America.[25]

While not mentioning Sweden by name, Eisenhower's remarks were picked up in Sweden and the other northern social democracies. Recognizing the caricature of his country, Tage Erlander (1901–85) – the Swedish prime minister at the time – dismissed the remarks, expressing amazement that Eisenhower had not taken the trouble to know what he was talking about when drawing his conclusions. On governmental paternalism, he said that the Swedish policy had been based on increasing the personal freedom of citizens. While Sweden did have its social problems, so did the USA.[26]

The conservative opposition in Sweden made the connection as well, and an editor of *Svenska Dagbladet* (*SvD*) expressed the view that it was difficult to recognize the Eisenhower view of Sweden, even by those Swedes who felt that the country could be more favourably disposed towards business. Fact-checking should have been carried out before offering criticism of social democracy.[27]

And the reading matter upon which Eisenhower had based his criticism of Sweden? Olof Palme (1927–86), then a member of Erlander's secretariat and a member of parliament, believed that writing by the American journalist Peter H. Wyden (1923–88) had been the source. Wyden had interviewed Erlander in the late-1950s and had asked questions pointing to the ambition of creating a controversial piece which would give Republicans the propaganda for the 1960 elections that could challenge Democrat welfare goals. The article ('*Sweden: paradise with problems*') had been published in the conservative and declining *Saturday Evening Post* in December 1959, and again in abridged form in the equally conservative *Reader's Digest* in March 1960.[28] Had the latter been Eisenhower's reading matter?

After he had left office, Eisenhower had arrived in Stockholm during a tour of Europe in 1962. Knowing that there was the possibility of a poor reception because of his remarks in 1960, he delivered a gracious apology at the very start of his visit dousing any protest that might have come his way. Relations between the two countries had not suffered any long-term damage, though these would deteriorate during the late-1960s and early-1970s – the Palme years – when the USA became militarily involved in south-east Asia, most graphically in Vietnam.[29]

The Palme Years – Shrill Criticism of Sweden – Totalitarian Welfare Dystopia

Palme had first awakened Swedish interest in distant Vietnam in a speech in Gävle in 1965, graphically and emotionally raising images of pain and torture, of mutilated children, and of crippled humanity. He had talked of acts of terrorism and reprisal (by the USA) that struck at individuals, families, and village communities in Vietnam. Then, in December 1972, after the American bombing of Hanoi and Haiphong, Palme's 'Christmas Speech' or '*Jultalet*' compared the aerial action to past atrocities in Guernica, Oradour, Babi Yar, Katyn, Lidice, Sharpeville, and Treblinka. In response, Richard Nixon, president since 1969, limited diplomatic contact with Sweden in a straining of relations.[30]

'Sweden-bashing' intensified again when Palme returned to power in 1982 after the brief non-socialist interregnum (1976–82). This time the criticism was not only evident in the USA but in western Europe too. In particular, the Swedish welfare state became the focus for persistent, intensive, and shrill criticism. Sweden was regarded as a welfare society in which the care of citizens had reached such levels as to be bordering on the totalitarian. In addition to economic difficulties and labour market conflict, foreign journalists eagerly reported on the high tax burden of Swedes, their effective bureaucracy and computerised social statistics which suggested state surveillance of the population, and to cap it all there was the personal identity number (*personnummer*).[31] Akin to a US social security number, or a UK national insurance number, an individual's personal identity number facilitated life in Sweden, giving its holder access to Swedish healthcare and social security. It was used in all contacts with Swedish authorities and agencies. But it wasn't just the personal identity number that irked.

In his book, *The new totalitarians* (1971), Roland Huntford, a correspondent writing on Scandinavia for the British press, launched a blistering polemic against Swedish social democracy. The thrust of his work which he later described as 'a youthful indiscretion, written with far too much emotion',[32] was that the political and social climate in Sweden at that time – the Social Democrats had been in power since the 1930s – resembled the dystopian state represented in Aldous Huxley's *Brave new world* (1931). His principal argument was that the Social Democratic government in Sweden relied less upon the violence and intimidation of the old 1930s European totalitarians to achieve its goals than upon soft persuasion and manipulation.

Huntford's work had been part of a wave of criticism of Sweden's welfare state that Gösta Grassman, a journalist and press officer at the Swedish foreign affairs ministry, would later describe as a new category of 'publicity' about Sweden – what the foreign ministry called 'the 1984 reports' – making a connection between the often-digressive narrative about Sweden and the totalitarian society of George Orwell's *Nineteen-eighty-four*.[33] The 'reports' offered nothing concrete and were most often based on anecdotes and vagueness, giving them a disproportionate impact because of the mental distance between the intended foreign audience and everyday Swedish life.[34]

Symbol of a Particular Way of Life

It was open to question whether Trump or Eisenhower had any interest in harming Sweden or the Swedes. Either way, they were both happy to sacrifice a chunk of goodwill from a small Nordic country on the altar of domestic politics.[35]

In 1960 and again in 2017, the most powerful men in the world had used Sweden as a symbol of a particular way of life that ought not to be followed and had used Swedish values as a set that ran contrary to their own.[36]

Eisenhower had made his comments just at the time when Sweden was being raised up as the perfect example of functioning socialism, having enjoyed uninterrupted growth since the war. It would have been no mean feat indeed for the president to have used the economic facts to argue that the Swedish model was failing. However, by implying that 'even Sweden' was plagued by drunkenness, lack of ambition and loose morals, he had a convenient emotional tool for associating that model with failure in the minds of Americans.[37]

Be they over rates of alcoholism, suicide, divorce, morality, crime, or migration, the fallout from vague accusations, unsupported argument, and from post-truth politics from American presidents, other national leaders and politicians, and journalists and the media, could stick and last a long time. And not least the claims of having 'most rapes per capita in the world', Sharia law in some areas of Sweden, and 'creeping Islamization', as offered respectively by Orbán, Hungarian prime minister, and Kaczyński, the leader of Poland's Law and Justice Party and a former prime minister, and Siv Jensen, the leader of the Norwegian Progress Party.[38] And so it was with COVID-19 and Sweden's approach to it – a country fixed in twenty-first century myth as 'outlier' just as it had been in the twentieth century.

In the contemporary world, Sweden appeared to have become a symbol in a larger political, economic, and moral context, mainly concerning the issue of migration, multiculturalism, and the right of asylum. Sweden also had symbolic value as a representative of a kind of progressive politics and openness, and it served as a positive model for many. As long as Sweden continued to perform comparatively well in most macroeconomic and social indicators, and at the same time strove to uphold human rights in its asylum policy, as well as freedom of expression, the country and its policies would continue to function, not least as a negative symbol in the US conservative worldview – a role in which it had served for so long.[39]

Sweden and COVID-19 – Argument in the Scientific Community

Then in 2020, along had come COVID-19, and more negativity, and into the mix had been thrown Sweden the exceptional, Sweden the superior, Sweden the 'outlier', Sweden the 'outrider', the country again lying well outside the normal range of behaviour.

From the outside world looking in, the Swedish approach to COVID-19 had become the 'infamous response' to the disease, and certainly not one to be followed. It amounted to a 'reckless or even murderous disregard'. For others, the Swedish approach had shown 'enlightened statecraft'.[40] For them, freedom-loving Swedes were supposedly pursuing a mask-free, lockdown-light strategy that would create herd immunity without bankrupting the economy. Sweden's approach had been successful and was a standing rebuke to those who wanted to shut everything down.[41]

Theories abounded as to why Sweden often behaved outside the normal range of behaviour. Attention and scrutiny became intense, and to help concoct an explanation, foreign journalists sought the input of Swedish colleagues, political scientists, epidemiologists, and other experts. Theorizing allowed writers to express a whole range of tropes and national characteristics – some negative, some positive, many cancelling out each other – to help explain the unique approach and to how Sweden had stood out. The end-product was a confused 'theory with everything' tying up the approach taken towards the coronavirus crisis in 2020 with the approach taken towards the migration crisis in 2015, with exceptionalism, moral superiority, neutrality, values, peacefulness, secularity, and rationality all thrown into the pot. And, just for good measure, there were the conflicting notions and anecdotes of Sweden in its 'little romantic world' where everything was fine, its collective high self-confidence, its improvisation and slow reaction and response, the strength of its state, its freedom-loving strategy, its being in the vanguard, and its being naïve. All of these were added to the mix, the whole thing shaken about a bit, and then thrown out again as an explanation.[42]

The intensity of the argument over infection control had become quite high, and in Carlson's opinion the number of experts in the field of infection control had also grown exponentially – almost at the same rate as the number of infections. It seemed that everyone was an expert, and this was a sense that he had experienced during the HIV epidemic in the very earliest years of his career. In the current debate about how best to tackle the spread of coronavirus, it had saddened him that the media had set loose so many experts who might indeed have been entitled to be labelled as such but had not done much research in this particular area.[43]

In the argument, the notion of a strategy to achieve herd immunity was returned to again and again by both detractors and supporters of the Swedish COVID-19 strategy. But for either side, this was a dead end. Sweden, in common with other countries, had simply been trying to slow down the spread as much as possible. To imply that Sweden was letting the disease run free without any measures to try to stop it was just not true.[44] Any reaching of herd immunity, or coming close to achieving it, would have been regarded as a by-product of other measures. Although Sweden had become a symbol of the debate around how to achieve population immunity, the goal had never been to suppress the virus entirely, but only to protect the national healthcare system and to make sure it could cope with COVID-19 while attending to the broader health of the population. Other countries had seemed ready to emulate Sweden at an early stage in the pandemic, not least the UK, but had caved in to public pressure as death tolls mounted.[45]

Anyway, what if achieving herd immunity had indeed been a formal component of Sweden's 'infamous response'? Wasn't it a respectable concept in epidemiology? Wasn't herd immunity the aim of mass vaccination programmes? Why was the concept of herd immunity loaded with such negativity? Was it maybe something to do with the negative way the word 'herd' had been applied to humans in philosophy and literature – the 'common herd', or 'herd mentality', or 'herd instinct', or 'herd minds' and so on?[46] Was it because by employing the word 'herd', humans were being classified as lumbering, uncomprehending cattle – mere followers? Was there something perhaps a bit dark – something Nazi and 1930s – about the term? What would happen to that part of the herd that was not immune? Where would they be taken?

Suggesting an approach grounded on herd immunity, and named after the town of Barrington in Massachusetts, USA, the Great Barrington Declaration authored 4 October 2020 by the epidemiologists and professors Kulldorff (Harvard), Gupta (Oxford), and Bhattacharya (Stanford), and supported by many other eminent co-signatories, proposed that the virus be allowed to spread freely among the younger and healthier of the population, while measures should be taken to protect the most vulnerable in it. Later, a rebuttal by epidemiologists, virologists, and other scientists and doctors – the John Snow Memorandum – was published in *The Lancet*, 14 October 2020, calling the Declaration a dangerous fallacy unsupported by scientific evidence. The Memorandum, named after physician John Snow (1813–58) who had established the principles of epidemiology, urged governments to do whatever it took to suppress the spread of the virus. It called for continued restrictions until testing, contact-tracing, and isolation systems were fixed and working properly.[47]

In the event, herd immunity in Sweden – by November 2020 at least – had been nowhere in sight. Back in April, the public health agency had predicted that 40 per cent of the population of Stockholm would have the disease, and by May would acquire protective antibodies. However, in September, the agency's own antibody studies showed that in samples taken up to late-June, the actual figure for random testing of antibodies was only 11.4 per cent for Stockholm, 6.3 per cent for Gothenburg, and 7.1 per cent across Sweden.[48]

And the UK? – 'Plague Island'

There was a certain calculation if not artifice in describing Sweden as an 'outlier' or 'outrider', and in painting its response as 'infamous', and an approach not to be emulated. Describing Sweden in these terms, and as a country 'doing nothing' to stop the spread of infection and giving disproportionate attention to criticism within Sweden of the Swedish strategy, diverted attention from failures and ineptitude in one's own country.

Could the Swedish approach have been emulated anyway? Depending on the audience being presented with this picture of Sweden – a UK audience for the sake of argument – an understanding would be required of the difference in dynamic between that audience and its government, and the dynamic existing in Sweden. There would have to be an understanding of the trust the Swedish population had in their government, and the greater individual responsibility taken by the average citizen, each of which were vital to the overall success of the Swedish approach in that high-trust society.

And the UK approach – could it be copied? While the Swedish strategy had its supporters, and New Zealand had ridden its storms with swift lockdowns, and Germany was escaping the worst through mass testing, no one was rushing to emulate the UK strategy. In spring 2020, during the first wave of COVID-19, a late lockdown brought the UK one of the highest recorded excess death rates in Europe. Over successive weeks of the pandemic, the UK suffered the worst economic recession of any of the G7.[49]

Facing a second wave in the autumn, the government of prime minister Boris Johnson again showed itself incapable of controlling the virus. On 21 September, the scientific advisory body SAGE (Scientific Advisory Group for Emergencies) produced a paper with the message that something had to be done now, or else control over the virus would be lost.[50] Rather than restricting social mixing, closing bars and pubs, and shifting university classes online, and advising working from home on the day the advice was given, Johnson ignored the science and procrastinated, and did not make a decision until 12 October.[51]

Coronavirus had laid bare Johnson's 'laziness, lack of focus, inflated triumphalist rhetoric, and flippant bonhomie'.[52] Towards the end of October, and because of delay and dither, the UK was facing the choice between a new national lockdown – a tiered system had fallen short of what SAGE had wanted in September – or thousands of additional deaths. In the end, on 31 October, Johnson proposed a new national lockdown in England, starting in November and lasting until early-December. After that, a tiered system would be in place, as in the other nations of the UK.

While some commentators had advocated following a strategy of herd immunity, others had suggested being a bit more like Sweden full-stop (Mark Woolhouse and the study and modelling carried out at the University of Edinburgh). However, the Swedish approach could not just be lifted wholesale and transposed to the UK. The import of a health model from abroad to cure the UK was a delusion. The Swedish strategy reflected the qualities for which the country had long been admired, namely: high levels of trust in one of the most equal societies in the world; an emphasis on child well-being; and a generous welfare state ensuring that individuals had the financial support needed for self-isolation. As far as the UK was concerned, it was the absence of these qualities that had intensified the coronavirus crisis: low levels of trust and mutual respect in one of the most unequal societies in the West; and high rates of child poverty and social deprivation. While Johnson's leadership had been inept, UK problems were of long-standing, and its injustices deep-rooted.[53]

Then there was Swedish governance too. The Swedish constitution gave the public health agency significant autonomy from government, with ministers expected to abide by its recommendations. The architect of the Swedish strategy had not been Löfven, the prime minister, but Tegnell who had led the agency since 2013.[54] No cabinet minister, not even the prime minister, had the power to intervene directly in a decision taken in the day-to-day agency's authority. Löfven and his cabinet – in collective decision-making – simply followed the science set before them. Johnson had delayed, dithered, and obfuscated when scientific advice was put before him.

In the last weeks of November, there would be renewed interest in the Swedish approach as a rash of measures were introduced that made the country seem more like the rest of Europe. The recalcitrant youth had put away his albums, turned down the volume, set aside teenage ways, and there could be heard a collective sigh of relief.

By December, and the approach to Christmas 2020, it was Johnson's UK that had begun to look like the 'outlier' or 'outrider', and the studiedly untidy, prime ministerial mop of blonde hair as ever seemed to reflect this. As the UK eagerly anticipated five days of relaxation of restrictions over the festival – but which some saw as a worrying scenario leading to an inevitable 'third wave' of the virus in January – the Netherlands was set to go into a strict lockdown for five weeks, with a slight easing for three days over Christmas itself. In Italy, a sober Christmas was expected, with many regions under partial lockdown, and a travel ban in place. In Germany, the Christmas period was to see a hard lockdown after a surge of deaths and infections in the weeks prior. Christmas Markets had already been cancelled and New Year fireworks displays too.[55]

In the event, the mutation of the coronavirus identified in the south-east of England in December, and the vastly increasing numbers of cases in London and the south-east, had brought an end to the planned relaxation. The UK found itself closed from the world as France, then country after country banned ferry, freight, and flights from the British Isles. The UK – Britain – had become 'plague island'.

Again the 'outlier' and buoyed up by its successful vaccination programme, in summer the following year, Johnson's UK – or England at least – had decided that 19 July 2021 would be 'freedom day', when legal COVID-19 restrictions would be lifted and the last remaining businesses would finally reopen. This was at a time when the more transmissible Delta-variant had become the dominant one across the country, and many younger people still had to be vaccinated. International experts had warned against the policy of ending social distancing and mask-wearing, warning that this would bring about 'herd immunity by mass infection'. Forging ahead towards unlocking was described as 'unscientific and unethical' and posed a 'danger to the world'. Official scientific advisors to the governments of Australia, Israel, Italy, and New Zealand, had all sounded alarm about the UK government strategy, fearing that such a reopening would allow the Delta-variant to spread rapidly around the world. England's chief medical officer, Professor Chris Whitty, had conceded that the number of those hospitalised with COVID-19 was doubling every three weeks.[56]

Moreover, by mid-July – as the unlocking approached – something like one third of the UK population had yet to receive one dose of vaccine. While 52.4 per cent of the UK population had received two doses, the share of people who had received one dose was 67.8 per cent.[57]

Statistics, July 2021 – Comparisons With UK, Larger European States

Meanwhile, the UK had been recording as many daily new cases per million as it had done in January 2021 – amounting to more than 50,000 per day. One of the country's scientific advisors, Professor Neil Ferguson who sat on the SAGE advisory group, said that the summer was going to be 'difficult' with cases 'almost certain' to reach 100,000 a day, with as many as 1,000 hospitalisations a day, and 'possibly' reaching 200,000 a day, with 2,000 hospital admissions a day – comparable to mid-January figures.[58]

Although it transpired that the scientists had miscalculated, statistics in high summer (mid-July 2021), showed that, of the larger European states – Russia, France, Germany, Italy, Spain, the UK, Ukraine – the UK had recorded 48,173 daily new confirmed COVID-19 cases (or 706.27 per million). Spain had recorded 27,688 (or 592.32 per million), Russia 24,793 (or 169.92 per million), France 11,042 (or 163.43 per million), Italy 2,473 (or 40.97 per million), Germany 1,444 (or 17.21 per million), and Ukraine 1,123 (or 25.84 per million).[59]

In October 2021, again only a few weeks away from Christmas, and even after an advanced and comprehensive vaccination programme, the UK had one of the highest rates of COVID-19 infection in Europe, registering some 50,000 cases on one day and more than Germany, France, Italy, and Spain combined.[60]

Just before Christmas at the end of the second year of the pandemic, the UK was again 'plague island'. As the Omicron-variant of COVID-19 took hold across the four nations of the UK – 10,000 of 78,000 cases had been of the new variant on one day alone – the French prime minister's office said that that the UK was going to face a landslide of Omicron. A week before Christmas, France tightened its COVID-19 restrictions for travellers arriving from the UK and they would have to have a compelling reason for doing so – tourism not being one of them. Skiing holidays in the Val D'Isere were out, as were Christmas breaks in 'Dordogneshire'.[61] A few days later, Germany followed France in banning most travellers from the UK. French and German nationals were of course still able to arrive home from the UK, and hauliers and transport workers were exempt.[62]

Chapter 7 focusses on the effects of the pandemic and the fight against it during the months of January to March 2021, paying particular attention to the Swedish and EU vaccination programmes and the first Swedish vaccinations, supply of vaccines, vaccine acceptance and resistance, vaccine passports and digital certificates, mutations and variants of the coronavirus, new restrictions and travel bans, and mask-wearing. Had Swedes been accepting of the vaccines? What about masks? The chapter also looks at the third wave of COVID-19 across Europe, the WHO report into the origins of the disease, and the possibilities for an international pandemic treaty.

Notes

1 O'Leary, Naomi. 'Sweden and coronavirus: how has the outlier of Europe fared?' *The Irish Times*, 23 September 2020, <https://www.irishtimes.com/news/world/europe/sweden-and-coronavirus-how-has-the-outlier-of-europe-fared-1.4362623> accessed 20 January 2022.

2 Ibid.

3 Ibid.

4 Milne, Robert. 'Sweden: why the moral superpower dissented over COVID-19', *Financial Times*, 16 October 2020, <https://www.ft.com/content/71c8a636-4d40-4d0e-947f-af8de9b6b82c> accessed 22 October 2020.

5 Ibid.

6 Ibid.

7 Simons, Gregg. 'Swedish government and country image during the international media coverage of the coronavirus pandemic strategy: from bold to pariah', p. 51, *Journalism and media*, 1 (1), pp. 41–58, Multidisciplinary Digital Publishing Institute, MDPI, published 12 November 2020, <https://doi.org/10.3390/journalmedia1010004> accessed 18 December 2021.

8 Irwin, Rachel Elisabeth. 'Misinformation and de-contextualization: international media reporting on Sweden and COVID-19', *Globalization and health*, 16, 2020, 13 July 2020, <https://globalizationandhealth.biomedcentral.com/articles/10.1186/s12992-020-00588-x#Sec9> accessed 18 December 2021.

9 Simons, as note 7, p. 53.

10 Irwin, as note 8, and, Bendjelloul, Johar. and Jonas Lindkvist. 'Folkhälsomyndighetens Johan Carlson: Det är klart att det kan kännas lite skrämmande', *Dagens Nyheter*, 5 April 2020, <https://www.dn.se/nyheter/sverige/folkhalsomyndighetens-johan-carlson-det-ar-klart-att-det-kan-kannas-lite-skrammande/> accessed 19 December 2021.

11 Ibid., Bendjelloul, and, Edwards, Catherine. 'Sweden's Anders Tegnell questioned over strategy and errors', *The Local*, 3 June 2020, <https://www.thelocal.se/20200603/swedens-anders-tegnell-questioned-over-strategy-and-errors> accessed 11 June 2020.

12 Simons, as note 7, p. 53.

13 Foster, Keith. 'US President Trump says Sweden is suffering in the corona crisis', *Sveriges Radio*, 11 April 2020, <https://sverigesradio.se/artikel/7450625> accessed 18 December 2021.

14 Foster, Alice. 'Sweden and Donald Trump: the controversy explained', *Express*, 20 February 2017, <https://www.express.co.uk/news/politics/769682/Sweden-Donald-Trump-controversy-explained-what-US-President-said-Swedish-incident> accessed 23 October 2020.

15 Ibid.

16 'Nation reacts to Trump's last night in Sweden comment', *Sveriges Radio*, 20 February 2017, <https://sverigesradio.se/sida/artikel.aspx?programid=2054&artikel=6635069> accessed 23 October 2020.

17 Eriksson, Aleksandra. 'Sweden fights back as foreign leaders make up bad news', eurobserver.com, 20 February 2017, <https://euobserver.com/nordic/136959> accessed 23 October 2020.

18 Ibid.

19 Christiansson, Magnus. 'Chapter II: The NATO question in Sweden under the Trump presidency - Military non-alignment between power politics and feminist foreign policy', p. 47, in *Finland, Sweden & Nato Did Trump Change Everything?* Edited by Jaan Siitonen / European Liberal Forum / Svenska Bildningsförbundet, Helsinki, 2017, pp. 39–55.

20 Brown, Joe David. 'Swedish sin', *Time* (Atlantic edition), 65, no.17, 25 April 1955, p.27.

21 Merklund, Carl. 'Därför beskrivs Sverige som en dystopi', *Dagens Nyheter*, 21 February 2017, <https://www.dn.se/kultur-noje/kulturdebatt/darfor-beskrivs-sverige-som-en-dystopi/> accessed 24 April 2020.

22 Hale, Frederick. 'Challenging the Swedish social welfare state: the case of Dwight D. Eisenhower', p. 57, *Swedish-American Historical Quarterly*, January 2003, v.54, no.1, pp.55-71. Films in question included the 1952 Palme d'Or nominated film *One summer of happiness* (Swedish title *Hon dansade en sommar*) directed by Arne Mattsson (1919–95) and starring Ulla Jacobsson (1929–82) and Folke Sundquist (1925–2009).

23 Bergan, Ronald. 'Petter Lindstrom', *The Guardian*, 17 June 2000, <https://www.theguardian.com/film/2000/jun/17/2/> accessed 24 April 2020. The 1953 film by Ingmar Bergman, *Summer with Monika* (*Sommaren med Monika*) starring Harriet Andersson was one of these featuring nudity. Sweden rapidly earned the reputation as a country 'with malleable standards of morality'

24 Orange, Richard. 'Muppets and free love: The bizarre documentary that shaped the image of Sweden', *The Local*, 12 March 2021, <https://www.thelocal.se/20210312/muppets-and-free-love-the-bizarre-documentary-that-shaped-the-image-of-sweden/> accessed 13 March 2021. Taboo films of the 1960s included: the 1963 Bergman film, *Tystnaden* (*The Silence*) starring Ingrid Thulin (1926–2004) and Gunnel Lindblom (1931–2021); the 1967 film *Jag är nyfiken–en film i gult* (*I am curious... Yellow*) directed by Vilgot Sjöman starring himself and Lena Nyman (1944–2011); then, the 1968 Italian film *Svezia, inferno e paradiso* (English title, *Sweden: Heaven and hell*), directed by Luigi Scattini.

25 Hale, as note 22, pp. 59–61.

26 Ibid., p. 61.

27 Ibid., pp. 61–62.

28 Ibid., p. 68.

29 Ibid., pp.67–69.

30 Merklund, Carl. 'From false neutrality to true socialism: US Sweden-bashing during the later Palme years, 1973-1986', *The journal of transnational American studies*, vol.7, issue 1, 2016.

31 Merklund, as note 21.

32 Crace, John. 'Out in the cold', an interview with Roland Huntford, *The Guardian*, 27 December 2008, <https://www,theguardian.com/books/2008/dec/27/interview-roland-huntford> accessed 25 April 2020.

33 Merklund, as note 30.

34 Merklund, as note 21. Another title in the 'report literature' genre was a book by Sture Källberg, *Off the middle way: Report from a Swedish village* (1972) which set out to portray the community of Västerås (then, more of a large town than a village, though doubtless that was the irony) through the lives of twelve of its inhabitants – farmers and workers. In an introduction to the book, Jan Myrdal (1927–2020), author, film-maker, and political activist, claimed that Källberg's work reflected a movement of cultural repossession. The title had served as a nod to the 1936 classic by Marquis Childs (1903–1990), *Sweden: The middle way*, an optimistic account of the path developed by Sweden between the extremes of capitalism and the fascism of the right and left, but according to a review by American sociologist, Norman Birnbaum (1926–2019), its content had given voice to Swedes who had 'lost their way' without a 'very clear idea of the reasons why'. The book had been less a description of modern Swedish society, said Birnbaum, and more 'a series of cries for help' (Birnbaum, Norman. 'Portrait of a Swedish town', *New York Times*, 24 September 1972).

35 Rapacioli, Paul. 'When a US president speaks about Sweden, the fallout can last a long time', *The Local*, offering an extract from Rapacioli's work *Good Sweden, bad Sweden* (Volante: Stockholm, 2018), 12 January 2018, <https://www.thelocal.se/20180112/how-swedens-good-reputation-is-being-challenged-by-ignorance> accessed 23 October 2020.
36 Ibid.
37 Ibid.
38 Eriksson, as note 17.
39 Merklund, as note 21.
40 Eaton, George. 'Trust is vital if you want to stop this disease', Anders Tegnell on leading Sweden's fight against Covid-19, p. 17 *New Statesman*, 23–29 October 2020, p. 16.
41 'Sweden and COVID-19. Land of the mask-free', *The Economist*, 10–16 October 2020, Vol. 437, No. 9215, p. 14.
42 Milne, as note 4.
43 Bendjelloul, as note 10.
44 Eaton, as note 40, p. 17.
45 Milne, as note 4.
46 Poole, Steven. 'Word of the week: who benefits from herd immunity', *The Guardian*, 14 October 2020, <https://www.theguardian.com/books/2020/oct/14/who-benefits-from-herd-immunity> accessed 24 October 2020.
47 'Science & technology. When doctors disagree', *The Economist*, Vol. 437, No. 9217, 24–30 October 2020, p. 77.
48 Habib, Heba. 'Covid-19: What Sweden taught Scandinavia for the second wave', *British Medical Journal, BMJ*, 27 November 2020, <https://doi.org/10.1136/bmj.m4456> accessed 30 November 2020.
49 'Lessons from the plague year', *New Statesman*, 23–29 October 2020, p. 3. The Group of Seven was made up of Canada, France, Germany, Italy, Japan, UK, and the USA.
50 Ibid.
51 Reicher, Stephen. 'Johnson has ignored the science and blown our chance to stop a second wave', *The Guardian*, 13 October 2020, <https://www.theguardian.com/commentisfree/2020/oct/13/johnson-ignored-science-second-wave-sage-advice> accessed 31 October 2020.
52 Ball, Philip. 'Ten lessons of the pandemic', p. 23, *New Statesman*, 23–29 October 2020, pp. 23–27.
53 *New Statesman*, 23–29 October 2020, as note 49.
54 Eaton, as note 40, p. 17.
55 'Coronavirus: How Europeans are preparing for Christmas and New Year', *BBC News*, 15 December 2020, <https://www.bbc.co.uk/news/world-europe-55058362> and, 'UK about to blunder into major Christmas error', *BBC News*, 15 December 2020, <https://www.bbc.co.uk/news/live/world-55313964> accessed 15 December 2020.
56 Forrest, Adam. 'Boris Johnson pursuing COVID policy of mass infection that poses danger to the world, scientists warn', *The Independent*, 16 July 2021, <https://www.indepdendent.co.uk/news/uk/politics/boris-johnson-covid-scientists-warning-b1885305.html> accessed 16 July 2021.
57 'Share of people who received at least one dose of COVID-19 vaccine, July 15, 2021', and, 'Share of the population fully vaccinated against COVID-19, July 15, 2021', Our World in Data, COVID-19 dataset, <https://ourworldindata.org> accessed 20 December 2021.
58 Shearing, Hazel. 'COVID: UK faces a difficult summer, says leading scientist', *BBC News*, 18 July 2021, <https://www.bbc.co.uk/news/uk-57877033> accessed 19 July 2021.
59 'Daily new confirmed COVID-19 case, July 15, 2021' & 'Daily new confirmed COVID-19 cases per million people, July 15, 2021', Our World in Data, COVID-19 dataset, <https://ourworldindata.org> accessed 20 December 2021.

60 Triggle, Nick. 'Covid: The UK is Europe's virus hotspot – does it matter?', *BBC News*, 9 October 2021, <https://www.bbc.co.uk/news/health-58849024> and, Picheta, Rob. 'The UK has more Covid-19 cases than France, Germany, Italy and Spain combined', CNN, 21 October 2021, <https://edition.cnn.com/2021/10/20/uk/uk-europe-covid-infections-cmd-gbr-intl/index.html> accessed 23 October 2021. On 21 October, the UK had recorded 51,548, while Germany had recorded 17,508, France 6,127, Italy 3,791, and Spain 1,881, making 29,307. The CNN report could well have added Serbia with 7,327 new cases, Belgium 6,239, and Poland 5,591 into the calculation and the combined figure would still have been less than 51,548 ('Daily new confirmed COVID-19 cases, October 21, 2021', Our World in Data, COVID-19 dataset, <https://ourworldindata.org> accessed 20 December 2021).

61 'COVID: France to drastically restrict travel from the UK', *BBC News*, 16 December 2021, <https://www.bbc.co.uk/news/world-europe-59679861> accessed 17 December 2021. The day referenced was Wednesday 15 December 2021.

62 Cursino, Malu. 'COVID: Germany tightens restrictions on UK travellers', *BBC News*, 20 December 2021, <https://www.bbc.co.uk/news/uk-59715820> accessed 20 December 2021.

The Fightback Had Begun

First Swedish Vaccinations – Indiscretions – Mutations and Variants – New Restrictions – Mask-Wearing

Sweden had recorded 8,727 deaths by the end of 2020, the first coronavirus year in Europe. Into 2021 however, the fightback had begun – the vaccination programme – and up to10 January and just past the Christmas and New Year festive season, 16,577 vaccine doses had been administered.[1]

On 15 January, the king and queen, aged 74 and 77 respectively, had been given vaccinations while staying at Stenhammar Palace in Södermanland where they had been in residence for most of the pandemic. This 'occasion' clearly set an example to Sweden's older generations, though uptake by the elderly across western Europe had generally been good anyway. Almost a year later, in January 2022, by which time the royal couple had received three vaccinations each, they both tested positive for COVID-19 and had mild symptoms. According to the rules, they had isolated themselves at home.[2]

Other measures would help in the fightback in addition to the vaccination programme, not least the wearing of face-coverings. In January, Johan Carlson, director-general of the public health agency, admitted making the 'embarrassing' mistake of travelling on a bus in Uppsala without a face-covering during rush hour, against the agency's own recommendation that coverings be worn. He had made the admission after being spotted at Stockholm Central railway station without a face-covering. In the subsequent media reporting about the station incident, Carlson had argued that the recommendations did not include station platforms or concourses so long as it was possible to keep a distance and then volunteered the information about the bus incident. While it was important to be a role model, he said, sometimes 'you forget, and it's human'.[3]

Meanwhile, as mutations of COVID-19 from the UK, South Africa, and Brazil showed greater virulence and rapid spread, countries were closing their borders and putting quarantine measures in place for travellers. 'Travel corridors' had been abandoned, and evidence of testing was required prior to entry. Over 25–26 January, the UK had passed a milestone 100,000 deaths, recording 98,610 on 25 January and 100,241 on 26 January.

In Sweden, the foreign ministry had warned that travellers should not be making unnecessary trips, but if they had to, they should keep informed about restrictions and on how the pandemic was developing. A general ban on travel to Sweden from non-EU/EEA countries had been put in place, except for those with Swedish nationality or residency, or those moving to live there, those working in key jobs, those coming for urgent family reasons. Some countries were exempt from the ban as well. Within the EU, it was possible to travel to Sweden from most member states, but not from Norway or Denmark (though again there were exemptions). Test and self-isolation applied to all travellers coming from the UK, South Africa, Brazil, and Norway, the latter of which saw its entire 1,600 km border with Sweden closed (and patrolled in places) for the first time since the Second World War.[4]

With the spreading of new mutations, and with the spread of infection still too high, the Swedish government wanted to limit the number of passengers travelling on long-distance trains and buses. Rail and bus operators were ordered to keep their seating capacity to only 50 per cent on journeys longer than 150 kilometres, and these restrictions would be in place from mid-February to end-May. The new measures would apply during the annual *sportslov* (the school winter sports break).[5] Meanwhile, the public health agency warned of an increase in cases, with possible reasons being low compliance with such recommendations as mask-wearing on public transport and working from home instead of commuting to a workplace.[6]

Other measures that the government wanted to apply would require legality, and under the framework of a new temporary Pandemic Law – giving extra powers to enact measures to curb the spread of COVID-19 – the government proposed a broader shutdown of society from March. The shutdown would include the closure of retail locations (excluding supermarkets and pharmacies and other essential businesses), gyms, swimming pools and other sports facilities, restaurants except for takeaways, and private event venues.[7] The Pandemic Law also gave municipalities the ability to ban people from certain outdoor spaces – squares, parks, beaches – if they believed there was a significant risk of crowding. The law would expire in September 2021.

In February, cases in the Stockholm Region had risen by 24.1 per cent, and there were worries that the country might be entering a third wave of COVID-19, a wave more serious than the second one in spite of the ongoing vaccination programme. In response, health authorities in Gothenburg and the Västra Götaland Region were urging people to wear face masks at all times on public transport, and not just during peak times. Meanwhile a cluster of the coronavirus Beta-variant first discovered in South Africa had been confirmed in Västmanland in central Sweden. By the last week of February, health authorities in Stockholm were also urging the wearing of face masks at all times, and across Sweden all restaurants and cafes were to close at 20.30, whether or not they sold alcohol.

As the world death toll from COVID-19 passed well over 2,000,000, Ann Linde, the Swedish foreign minister announced in February that Sweden had contributed SEK 200 million to the COVAX global vaccination initiative, and that this contribution was part of some EUR 853 million mobilised by the EU.

To secure supplies for EEA countries, in February Sweden had undertaken to sell vaccines on to Norway, Iceland, and Switzerland.[8]

Statistics, March 2021 – Anniversary of First Swedish Death

On 11 March 2021, Sweden passed a sad milestone in its COVID-19 history. This had been the anniversary of the country's first recorded death from the infection – the victim having been a 70-year-old woman at the Karolinska University Hospital in Huddinge, Stockholm. On the anniversary, 11 March 2021, Sweden had recorded 13,111 deaths.

11 March 2020 had also been the day that the WHO declared the outbreak to be a global pandemic. A year later, across the world there had been 2.71 million deaths, and of these 849,760 had occurred in Europe, 570,518 in the EU, just under 2,400 in Denmark, around one fifth of the Swedish total, 776 in Finland, 639 in Norway, and 29 in Iceland.[9]

Royal Coronavirus Cases – Prime Minister Gives Admonishment

Also in March, the king's eldest daughter and son-in-law, crown princess Victoria and prince Daniel, both tested positive for COVID-19 after developing cold symptoms.

They had gone into quarantine with their children, princess Estelle and prince Oscar, and contact-tracing had been carried out. Earlier, in November 2020, the brother and sister-in-law of the crown princess – Carl Philip and Sofia – had both tested positive to COVID-19.[10]

At a press conference in March, at the same time as giving a statement on the Oxford/AstraZeneca vaccine and the need for public confidence in it, Stefan Löfven had said that infection rates were now at much too high a level and he had given what amounted to a stern admonishment to those not following the recommendations that were in place. More and more people were ignoring the advice and recommendations, and this was having an effect on the spread of infection. People needed to do more, for the country and for the good of everyone, he said. Big Easter family celebrations in Sweden were out of the question, he had added. COVID-19 did not care about festivities. Carlson had also been present at the press conference, and when asked if the decision to keep Swedish ski resorts open, and failing to advise against travelling during the winter *sportlov* holiday, had contributed to the rising infection rate, he said it was too early to tell, though there was nothing to suggest that it had.[11] The prime minister's admonishment had come only a few months after the death of his foster-mother.

Later, Anders Tegnell the state epidemiologist had offered more clarity when he said that, based on infection rates in and around mountain resorts, the holiday had no effect whatsoever. He had added that, according to analysis carried out in Region Skåne, the spread of infection had been higher among those staying at home than those who had spent time in mountain holiday resorts.

Swedish and EU Vaccination Programmes – Efficacy of Oxford/AstraZeneca Vaccine Questioned – Problems With Production and Supply – EU Unity Evaporates

At the start of the year, some countries were accused of expressing 'vaccine nationalism' and waging 'vaccine wars' as supplies of vaccination doses to the EU became an issue.

In Germany, questions were raised over the efficacy of the Oxford/AstraZeneca vaccine in the over 65s, and the Pfizer/BioNTech (US-German developed) vaccine was profiled in preference.

In France, the president, Emmanuel Macron, claimed that the Oxford/AstraZeneca hadn't worked 'as expected' and was 'quasi-ineffective' in the over 65s. Outrage broke out in the UK as the EU sought to 'control the export of vaccines' and there were fears that it would try to hold back the Belgian-made Pfizer vaccine in retaliation for AstraZeneca refusing to divert supplies to the EU from its UK plants.[12]

Then, in February, the public health agency in Sweden also declared that it believed there was a lack of evidence for the efficacy of the Oxford/AstraZeneca vaccine among the over 65s. Approved vaccines from Pfizer/BioNTech and Moderna should be offered to over 65s instead. The change would of course bring delays to the Swedish vaccination programme.[13]

In addition to the question of efficacy, the supply and production of vaccine had presented the EU with difficulties. In early-February, Ursula von der Leyen admitted that the EU had been late in authorising COVID-19 vaccines and was still not where it wanted to be in the rollout. She had also acknowledged that the EU had been over-confident about production targets.[14] While in December 2020, von der Leyen had talked of a touching moment of unity when the EU vaccine rollout began, by March 2021 the EU vaccination programme was sluggish if not stuttering, with claims of unfair distribution of vaccines across member states, and that a number of them had reached side deals with manufacturers. EU unity appeared to have evaporated.

Evidence of a fraying of unity had been shown by Austria and Denmark when they began coordinating with Israel on developing new vaccines (second generation vaccines), and when Sebastian Kurz, the Austrian Chancellor, criticised the European Medicines Agency (EMA) for being too slow in approving vaccines. As central Europe began registering a third wave of the virus, Hungary and Czechia would also seek discussions with Israel. Slovakia, Hungary, and Czechia had already bypassed the EMA to approve Russian and Chinese vaccines, while France had criticised attempts at secession from the EU programme. Meanwhile, Hans Kluge, European Director of WHO, talked of the resurgence of COVID-19 across Europe, especially in central and eastern Europe.[15]

Against the background of criticism of the slowness of rollout, Italy had blocked an export of vaccine to Australia in March, stating that there was a lack of urgent need in Australia and a shortage of vaccine across Europe. Von der Leyen warned that the EU could halt further exports of vaccine.[16]

She also said that four million extra vaccine doses would be deployed to COVID-19 hotspots, particularly to badly affected border regions so that virus-related border restrictions could be lifted to ensure or restore free movement of goods and people. A steep rise in infection in the Austrian Tyrol, the French Nice and Moselle regions, the area around Bolzano in Italy, and in the German regions of Bavaria and Saxony, had led to the application of strong measures and controls in these border areas. For the EU Commission, restoring freedom of movement within the EU was key to the functioning of health systems and the single market.[17]

Later in March, the EU had tightened its vaccine export control mechanism – introducing reciprocity and proportionality before authorizing exports – to prevent an unfair flow of vaccines outside of its borders. This would likely limit exports to the UK, for example, which produced some of its own vaccines, but did not send doses to the EU.[18]

Despite delayed deliveries of the Pfizer/BioNTech and Moderna vaccines, Sweden claimed that it still expected to offer a coronavirus vaccine to its entire adult population by the end of June, though authorities in Stockholm did not expect to achieve that target before mid-July. By mid-February only 1.65 per cent of people in Sweden had been fully vaccinated (the initial two-dose protocol) relative to population. In the EU 1.7 per cent had been fully vaccinated, and in the UK 0.8 per cent. In Denmark the figure was 2.7 per cent, in Iceland 1.6 per cent, Norway 1.4 per cent, and in Finland 1.3 per cent. The actual numbers fully vaccinated were, in the UK 539,630, in Sweden 167,665, in Denmark 157,131, in Norway 75,856, in Finland 69,904, and in Iceland 5,757. By mid-March, statistics showed that 3.8 per cent of people had been fully vaccinated in Sweden (the initial two-dose protocol) relative to population, while in the EU it was 3.6 per cent, and in the UK 2.6 per cent. In Norway the figure was 5 per cent, in Denmark 4.5 per cent, in Iceland 3.7 per cent, and in Finland 1.6 per cent. The actual numbers fully vaccinated were, in the UK 1.76 million, in Sweden 385,247, in Norway 272,566, in Denmark 263,079, in Finland 89,202, and in Iceland 13,552.[19]

If Sweden managed to stick to its timetable, the population might manage to enjoy part of the summer in a social environment close to 'normal'. As it turned out however, by end-March 2021 when only 5 per cent of the adult population had been fully vaccinated, it looked like Sweden was not going to achieve the goal of vaccinating the entire adult population by the end of June. At the end of April, it was 8 per cent fully vaccinated, at the end of May, 15 per cent, and at the end of June, 31 per cent. At mid-July, when the authorities had expected to achieve the target of a fully vaccinated adult population, the actual share of people vaccinated was still only 38 per cent, or 3.86 million people.[20]

'Vaccination Passports' and 'Digital Certificates'

In early-February, the government had instructed Lena Hallengren, the health and social affairs minister, Anders Ygeman, the digitalisation minister, and Carlson at the public health agency, to work on a digital vaccination certificate in time for the summer.

This optional 'vaccination passport' would be used to prove that the holder had been vaccinated and to facilitate travel abroad. The digital infrastructure would be put together to make vaccination certification more secure, simple, and international. Denmark had already announced plans for the rollout of vaccination passports.[21] The EU had also laid out plans for an EU-wide pass to facilitate travel, proving either vaccination or recent testing for those not yet vaccinated.

The EU plan for what was being described as a 'digital certificate' had been unveiled in mid-March, with the hope that it would help reinstate freedom of movement in a safe, responsible, and trusted manner. It would show, said von der Leyen, whether a person had either been vaccinated or had a recent negative test, or had recovered from COVID-19, and had antibodies. The plan however was likely to face resistance in some member states because of fears of discrimination against those still awaiting vaccination, indeed programmes across the EU had been patchy. Additionally, the WHO had warned that there was no evidence to show that those who had recovered from COVID-19, and who had antibodies, were protected from a second infection.[22] As of mid-March, only 3.6 per cent of the European population had been fully vaccinated (had received the requisite doses needed).

New COVID-19 Variants Dominant in Sweden – New Travel Bans

By mid-March, Sweden's vaccination programme had contributed to a continuing week-on-week decline in newly reported deaths from COVID-19.

However, a briefing from Tegnell said that there was an increasing presence of the new variants of the coronavirus in Sweden. The Alpha-variant had been present in more than 50 per cent of positive tests analyzed across thirteen regions, and the Beta and Gamma variants had been discovered in more than 10 per cent of tests in four regions (the Gamma-variant had arisen in the Amazonas state of Brazil). A ban had been put in place against travel from the UK, Denmark, and Norway, and all travellers regardless of the country travelled to had to isolate and avoid close contacts for at least seven days after arriving in Sweden. They also had to get tested twice, once on arrival, and the second five days after. The bans against travel from Denmark and Norway would be in place until end-March.[23]

These had been timely requirements, because later in March, Tegnell had announced a further increase in cases and new pressures on Sweden's hospitals and ICUs. The assessment of the public health agency was that the increased spread was due to declining compliance with existing recommendations and restrictions.[24]

Blood Clots and the Oxford/AstraZeneca Vaccine

March brought renewed spotlight on the Oxford/AstraZeneca vaccine, and a new round of problems for vaccination programmes across the EU.

Sweden had suspended the Oxford/AstraZeneca vaccination from its programme over fears of blood clots from the product, although Denmark, then Iceland and Norway, had been the first to implement a suspension. Ireland and the Netherlands, then Bulgaria, Austria, France, Germany, and Italy, and several other countries across the EU, had followed suit. The WHO said that while investigations were carried out, people should continue having their vaccinations, and the EMA said that there had been no indication that the vaccine had caused thrombotic events in people who had been vaccinated. Confirmation in a report from the EMA that the Oxford/AstraZeneca could be safely used came a few days later, and some countries began their programmes again, though Denmark, Norway, and Sweden would wait until the own relevant agencies had given the go-ahead.

Towards the end of March, Germany paused the use of the Oxford/AstraZeneca vaccine for the under-60s, despite EMA assurances. The chancellor, Angela Merkel, had told journalists that the advice had been prompted by the occurrence of rare but very serious cases of thrombosis among younger and predominantly female recipients of the vaccine. Meanwhile, Canada had suspended its use in the programme for under-55s.[25]

In Sweden, Löfven said that what was most important was for the public to be fully confident that the safety risks had been properly evaluated, and that everyone felt safe when they got their vaccination. Carlson said that they needed time to digest what the EMA had said in their full report.[26] Later on in March, the agency announced a restart of the programme using the Oxford/AstraZeneca vaccine, but only for the over-65s. Denmark and Finland had also resumed rollout of the vaccine for over-65s.

The question was: Had European governments been wrong to suspend their vaccination programmes? After all, there had been a huge risk that pausing the programme would cause resistance among the public towards vaccines and reduce vaccine acceptance.

Side Effects and Vaccine Acceptance – Public Resistance

When vaccination programmes moved beyond the vulnerable groups, and health and care workers, and began targeting the wider public, countries with high vaccine acceptance had the advantage and started to make progress against infection. Traditionally, Sweden had shown high acceptance of vaccines, and for its normal child vaccination programme, and set of vaccines against a battery of preventable diseases, the uptake had been 97 per cent.[27] In lockdown countries however, when all action had been focussed on COVID-19, other health interventions suffered. Globally, in 2021, some 25 million children missed out on childhood vaccinations – the biggest drop in thirty years. In Sweden, there had been no drop at all.[28]

As far as COVID-19 was concerned, among Swedish elderly, a willingness to get vaccinated would probably remain high since they had so much to gain. Among the younger age groups however, willingness to get vaccinated was likely to be lower than expected. It would take only a small increase in the number of people unwilling to get vaccinated to make it difficult to achieve herd immunity, especially as the more infectious Alpha-variant was becoming dominant in Sweden. Joakim Dillner, a professor in infectious disease epidemiology at the Karolinska University Hospital, had said that it would require 75 per cent of the population to be vaccinated to reach herd immunity, but with the new variant it would need up to 85 per cent.[29]

At the same time, letting the vaccination programmes continue in the face of evidence of rare clotting cases in several different countries could have had a calamitous effect on public attitudes. Governments faced being damned if they did, and damned if they did not. Among the media in the UK, the prevalent view was that EU countries were engaging in 'vaccination nationalism', or simply being stupid, attacking the Oxford/AstraZeneca vaccine on flimsy pretext. It was all political, they said. However, the opposite was the case. Decisions across Europe had been taken based on medical and legal considerations, and political interests had given way to these.[30]

Belgium had gone against that trend, courageously, and had not suspended its AstraZeneca vaccination programme, saying that to do so would have been irresponsible. Thousands of lives would be saved by the vaccine, while only a handful 'might' be lost through very rare side effects. The Belgian decision did not make other countries irresponsible. While it was asserted in the UK that there had been no connection between the Oxford/AstraZeneca vaccine and clotting disorders, and that the thromboses had been less common among those having had the vaccine than in the general population, neither of these assertions had been true. Norwegian research found that there was a link between the vaccine and three cases of rare brain thromboses that had occurred in Norway, and in Germany there had been seven cases of cerebral venous sinus thrombosis (CVST) among 1.6 million Germans who had been given the vaccine – four times higher than the normal rate. Shouting down understandable caution – as the UK had done – was foolish and hazardous. Reviewing the evidence, as European governments were doing, had been sensible.[31]

Their actions would be justified in early-April when the EMA gave a revised opinion, saying that a link between the Oxford/AstraZeneca vaccine and clotting did exist. Its safety committee – the Pharmacovigilance Risk Assessment Committee, PRAC – concluded that 'unusual blood clots with low blood platelets' should be listed as 'very rare' side effects of the vaccine, now being referred to as Vaxzevria. The EMA would be reminding healthcare professionals and recipients of the vaccine to remain aware of the possibility of very rare cases occurring within two weeks of vaccination. The fact also remained that the overall benefits of Vaxzevria in preventing COVID-19 outweighed the risks of side effects.[32]

Europe and the Third Wave

With a third wave of the virus already striking central Europe – a wave given added force by more contagious and more deadly variants – other countries began tightening their restrictions once again into late-March.

In Germany and France, night curfews would be put in place, and France had brought in regionalized 'lockdown-light' restrictions. Italy had placed around half of the country into a medium-risk 'orange' zone, and the remainder in a higher-risk 'red' zone. In the orange zone, people were not allowed to leave their own towns except for urgent reasons, while in the red zone people had to stay in their own homes except for fetching essentials. In Norway, local and national restrictions were put in place including a ban on the serving of alcohol and on organized sporting and leisure activities for adults. In addition, everyone returning to Norway after foreign travel had to isolate in a quarantine hotel for ten days. Over Easter 2021, all non-essential travel was to be avoided. In Austria and Switzerland, lockdowns were to be in place until after Easter. An extended lockdown was in place in the Netherlands too.[33]

In Denmark though, restrictions previously put in place were beginning to be eased. Schools were partially open, and smaller shops were reopening too, though entertainment venues and restaurants remained closed. The majority of restrictions were to be lifted once everyone over the age fifty had been vaccinated – perhaps by May. In Spain too there had been an easing of restrictions, and in the four nations of the UK schools had re-opened and pubs were set to open outdoor service in April. By June, it was possible that all limits on social contact would be lifted across the UK.[34]

Iceland Reopens

While much of the rest of Europe was in lockdown again in March, Iceland had virtually rid itself of COVID-19.

The island nation had become Europe's only 'green' country in the 'traffic light system' that had been adopted between June and October 2020. Concerts were happening, restaurants and night venues were open again, hugging and kissing was 'allowed', and there was only a handful of active coronavirus cases with just one in hospital. In total, Iceland had recorded 29 deaths (85 per million).[35]

Iceland had reached that milestone before however, having declared itself COVID-free by May 2020. The chief epidemiologist, Þórólfur Guðnason (Thorolfur Gudnason) had been placed firmly in charge of the country's response to the pandemic from the very beginning, with politicians taking a backseat and absent from daily briefings. Testing, contact-tracing, and isolation of everyone diagnosed had been put in place immediately, and followed aggressively, in preparations that Guðnason had been planning over fifteen years. Iceland had also benefitted from the use of the state-of-the-art laboratories of biopharmaceutical company deCODE genetics, handed over by Kári Stefánsson the founder of the company when COVID-19 hit the island. Despite these advantages however, in summer 2020 the country had been hit by a second and unexpectedly ferocious wave of the virus after two tourists testing positive had broken isolation rules. From June, every arriving passenger would be put through quarantine and there would be mandatory testing at the airport.[36]

Iceland and its politicians – led by a red-green government headed by Katrín Jakobsdóttir of the Left-Green Movement (*Vinstrihreyfingin – grænt framboð*) – had followed the science. Politicians had listened to the experts and understood the difference between politics and what needed to be solved scientifically. Getting behind the programme of rigorous testing, contact-tracing, and isolation, the country had managed to stop the Alpha-variant taking a grip by containing cases at the border.[37]

WHO Report – Global Study of the Origins of SARS-CoV-2

Towards the end of March, the outcome of research and fact-finding on the other side of the world from Iceland had been released. This was the final report of the WHO-convened global study into the origins of SARS-CoV-2, or COVID-19, conducted in Wuhan, China, between 14 January and 10 February 2021.

The study had been carried out by an international team of epidemiologists, data scientists, laboratory experts, food safety experts, veterinary epidemiologists, and animal health experts. The team was composed of seventeen Chinese members, and seventeen international members, and was headed jointly by Dr Peter K. Ben Embarek, Monitoring Nutritional Status and Food Safety Events, Nutrition and Food Safety, at the WHO, and Professor Liang Wannian of the Vanke School of Public Health, Tsinghua University. The team also included two observers from the Food and Agricultural Organization (FAO).[38]

The team had concluded that the most likely pathway for SARS-CoV-2 into the human population had been through direct zoonotic spillover (transmission of microorganisms from wild animals to humans), from bats, and that introduction through an intermediate animal host, pangolins, was also to considered likely. Surveys and targeted studies had shown that the coronaviruses most related to SARS-CoV-2 were found in bats and pangolins suggesting that these mammals might be the reservoir of the virus causing COVID-19. The team found that while many of the early cases of the virus were associated with the Huanan Seafood Wholesale Market in Wuhan, a similar number of cases were associated with other markets, and some were not associated with any markets. No firm conclusion about the role of the Huanan market in the origin of the outbreak, or how the infection was introduced into the market, could currently be drawn. In addition, data from different countries suggested early circulation of SARS-CoV-2, and that circulation of the virus preceded the initial detection of cases by several weeks. Some positive samples had been detected even earlier than the first case in Wuhan, suggesting the possibility of missed circulation in other countries.[39]

The team also found that supply chains to Huanan market included cold-chain products and animal products from twenty countries, including those where samples had been reported as positive for SARS-CoV-2 before the end of 2019, and those where close relatives of SARS-CoV-2 had been found. But, due to a lack of awareness of the potential role of the cold chain in virus introduction and transmission in the earliest phase of the pandemic, chilled/frozen products had not been tested. This raised the possibility of different potential pathways of introduction. SARS-CoV-2 had been found to persist in conditions found in frozen food, packaging and cold chain products, and the virus had been found on packages and products from other countries that supplied China with cold chain products, indicating that it could be carried long distances on these products.[40]

Finally, the team assessed as an extremely unlikely pathway the introduction of COVID-19 through a laboratory incident in Wuhan.[41] Such a conclusion would show however to be completely at odds with the later findings of the US House Select Subcommittee on the Coronavirus Pandemic. In its final report nearly four years later, December 2024, entitled *After action report of the COVID-19 pandemic: The lessons learned and a path forward*, the subcommittee found that 'COVID-19 most likely emerged from a laboratory in Wuhan, China', with five strong arguments in favour of the 'lab leak' theory.[42]

An International Pandemic Treaty?

The WHO report had been published just as political leaders around the world were calling for a new global settlement on future pandemics in a joint article released on 30 March 2021 through major newspaper titles – *Le Monde*, *El Pais*, and *The Telegraph*.

The COVID-19 pandemic had probably been the greatest challenge to the world since the Second World War. From 1945 and into the 1950s, political leaderships had come together to rebuild the international system, and to create institutions – namely the UN, NATO, and the foundation body that would eventually become the EU – that would confront isolationism and nationalism with a spirit of solidarity and cooperation.[43] In 2021, the same hope was held for a global effort to overcome COVID-19, and to build a more robust international health architecture.

The world had to be better prepared to predict, prevent, detect, assess, and respond effectively to pandemics in a more coordinated way. COVID-19 had been a reminder that nobody was safe until everyone was safe. Universal and equitable access to safe, effective, and affordable vaccines, medicines, and diagnostics for this and future pandemics had to be ensured. This had been the motivation behind the Access to COVID-19 Tools Accelerator (ACT-A), which had been set up to promote equal access to tests, treatments, and vaccines, and to support health systems around the world. While ACT-A had delivered – and the COVAX initiative was an example – there was more that could be done.[44]

Together with Dr Tedros Adhanom Ghebreyesus, director-general of the WHO, and Charles Michel, president of the European Council, some two dozen world leaders declared that the nations of the world should work together towards a new international treaty for pandemic preparedness and response. They included Mario Draghi, the Italian prime minister, Uhuru Kenyatta, the Kenyan president, Angela Merkel, the German chancellor, Mark Rutte, the Dutch prime minister, Erna Solberg, the Norwegian prime minister, Joko Widodo, the Indonesian president, and other world leaders from the UK to Fiji, from Romania to Senegal, and from France to Chile. This renewed collective commitment would be grounded in the constitution of the WHO, drawing in other relevant organisations. The principal goal of the treaty would be to encourage 'an all-of-government and all-of-society approach' to strengthen national, regional, and global capacities and resilience to future pandemics.[45]

Recognizing that neither individual governments nor the global community could entirely prevent pandemics, the proposal for an international treaty was first announced by Michel, at the Paris Peace Forum in November 2020. The call had also been highlighted by the G7 leaders in their statement on 19 February 2021, and EU leaders agreed to work on a treaty on 25 February 2021.[46]

A special provision of the WHO constitution, under Article 19, empowered the World Health Assembly (the decision-making body of the WHO) to negotiate and agree on 'conventions and agreements with respect to matters within the competence of WHO'. The article had been used in 2003 for the adoption of the framework convention on tobacco control. The treaty on pandemics would likely be adopted by the WHO member states gathering at the World Health Assembly (WHA).[47] The 74th WHA had been scheduled for 24 May–1 June 2021.

Swedish Responses to the Global Task

While Löfven the Swedish prime minister was not among the political leaders calling for an international pandemic treaty, neither had the leaders of Australia, Canada, nor New Zealand, nor Joe Biden in the USA, nor Vladimir Putin in Russia, nor the leaders of Denmark, Finland, and China been among them.

That did not mean that Sweden was not standing up in support of international principles and commitments, and in support of multilateral organisations working to fight the pandemic and its impacts. Rather, its work and ambitions were in line with the UN 2030 Agenda. Sweden's allocation of 1 per cent of GDP to development assistance was well known, and through international development cooperation it was contributing directly and indirectly to the fight against COVID-19. Swedish support was aimed towards building resilience in the health systems of low- and middle-income countries, and to increasing access to vaccines, diagnostics, treatments, and mitigating the socio-economic impacts of the pandemic.[48]

In addition to core support to international funds, programmes and organisations, Sweden allocated SEK 1.86 billion to COVID-19-specific support in 2020, and SEK 673 million towards addressing indirect consequences of the pandemic, mainly humanitarian assistance. This had included an initial grant of SEK 100 million to COVAX (the facility for access to COVID-19 vaccines by low- and middle-income countries). In 2020, Sida (the Swedish International Development Corporation Agency) had allocated some SEK 1.5 billion for COVID-19-support, which was around 6 per cent of its total disbursements. Much of the money was for the support of social infrastructure, health, sexual and reproductive health and rights, and humanitarian assistance, as well as support to governments and civil society and access to energy, water, and sanitation.[49]

Carl Bildt, Special ACT-A Envoy

On 31 March 2021, Ghebreyesus had appointed former Swedish foreign minister and prime minister Carl Bildt as WHO special envoy for the ACT-A which had been launched almost a year previously. His role would be to help lead 'collective advocacy' for the ACT-A, mobilising support and resources for the delivery of its strategy.[50]

Bildt would be joining the ACT-A at a crucial time when, around the world, vaccine programmes were underway, new diagnostics were being introduced, and treatments for severe disease were being scaled up, and while the uneven distribution of vaccines was being addressed. His role would support co-convening agencies, especially in work that cut across diagnostics, therapeutics, vaccines, and health systems.[51]

Chapter 8 examines the pandemic between April and July 2021, looking at renewed lockdowns, the WHO call to ban live animal sales in food markets, anxiety over blood clots, rising infection rates, the onslaught of the virus in India, and May Day protests in Sweden. It then describes the reopening of Sweden alongside the ongoing vaccination programme, the decline in coronavirus cases overall, and the arrival of the Delta-variant. Was the vaccination programme reaching everyone?

Notes

1 ‘Covid-19 vaccine doses administered, January 10, 2021’, Our World in Data, COVID- 19 dataset, <https://ourworldindata.org> and, ‘Vaccinering mot covid-19 inleds den 27 december’, Socialdepartementet, Regeringskansliet, <https://www.regeringen.se/artiklar/2020/12/vaccinering-mot-covid-19-inleds-den-27-december/> accessed 13 January 2022.

2 ‘King and queen of Sweden test positive for COVID-19’, *The Local*, 4 January 2022, <https://www.thelocal.se/20220104/king-and-queen-of-sweden-test-positive-for-covid-19/> accessed 5 January 2022.

3 ‘Embarrassing: Sweden’s public health chief rode the bus without a mask’, *The Local*, 28 January 2021, <https://www.thelocal.se/20210128/embarrassing-swedens-public-health-chief-used-public-transport-without-a-face-mask> accessed 28 January 2021.

4 ‘What are the rules on travel into Sweden?’ *The Local*, 25 January 2021, <https://www.thelocal.se/20210125/what-are-the-rules-on-travel-into-sweden-coronavirus-test-quarantine-isolation> and, ‘In pictures: Sweden closes 1,600 kilometre border with Norway’, *The Local*, 26 January 2021, <https://www.thelocal.se/20211226/in-pictures-sweden-closes-1600-kilometre-border-with-norway> accessed 26 January 2021.

5 ‘50 percent rule: Bid to force Swedish trains to cut passenger numbers’, *The Local*, 9 February 2021, <https://www.thelocal.se/20210209/50-percent-rule-bid-to-force-trains-to-cut-passenger-numbers> accessed 10 February 2021.

6 ‘Sweden’s Public Health Agency warns fewer people are following COVID-19 recommendations’, *The Local*, 16 February 2021, <https://www.thelocal.se/20210216/swedens-public-health-agency-warns-fewer-people-are-following-covid-19-recommendations/> 17 accessed 2021.

7 Edwards, Catherine. ‘Explained: The five new coronavirus measures that Sweden just announced’, *The Local*, 17 February 2021, <https://www.thelocal.se/20210217/explained-the-five-new-coronavirus-measures-annonced-by-sweden> accessed 17 February 2021.

8 Statement of Government Policy by Minister for Foreign Affairs, Ann Linde, in the Parliamentary Debate on foreign affairs, Wednesday 24 February 2021, Government Offices of Sweden, p. 1.

9 ‘Cumulative confirmed COVID-19 deaths, March 11, 2021, Our World in Data, COVID-19 dataset, <https://ourworldindata.org> accessed 13 January 2022.

10 ‘Sweden’s Crown Princess Victoria tests positive for COVID-19’, *The Local*, 11 March 2021, <https://www.thelocal.se/20210311/swedens-crown-princess-victoria-tests-positive-for-covid-19/> accessed 17 March 2021.

11 ‘Swedish PM: People are getting lazy in following the Covid-19 recommendations’, *The Local*, 19 March 2021, <https://www.thelocal.se/20210319/swedish-pm-people--covid-recommendations-astrazeneca-vaccine/> accessed 21 March 2021.

12 Yorke, Harry. and Lucy Fisher, Sarah Knapton, James Crisp. ‘Fury at Emmanuel Macron’s nonsense claims about Oxford Covid vaccine’, *The Telegraph*, 29 January 2021, <https://www.telegraph.co.uk/politics/2021/01/29/fury-macrons-attack-oxford-jab/> accessed 30 January 2021.

13 ‘Sweden recommends AstraZeneca vaccine only for people aged under 65’, *The Local*, 2 February 2021, <https://www.thelocal.se/20210202/sweden-recommends-astra-zeneca-covid-vaccine-only-for-people-aged-under-65> accessed 2 February 2021.

14 ‘Covid: EU’s von der Leyen admits vaccine rollout failures’, *BBC News*, 10 February 2021, <https://www.bbc.co.uk/news/world-europe-56009251> accessed 16 February 2021.

15 ‘Covid-19 cases in Europe back on the rise after weeks of decline’, *The Local*, 4 March 2021, <https://www.thelocal.se/20210304/covid-19-cases-in-europe-back-on-the-rise-after-weeks-of-decline/> accessed 4 March 2021, and, ‘Visiting Israel, leaders of Denmark, Austria agree

on joint vaccine development', *Times of Israel*, 4 March 2021, <https://www.timesofisrael.com/visiting-israel-leaders-of-denmark-austria-agree-on-joint-vaccine-development> accessed 5 May 2025.

[16] 'EU warns it could block more vaccine exports', *The Local*, 9 March 2021, <https://www.thelocal.se/20210309/eu-warns-it-could-block-more-vaccine-exports/> accessed 17 March 2021.

[17] 'Europe's Covid-19 hotspots to be sent four million more vaccine doses', *The Local*, 10 March 2021, <https://www.thelocal.se/20210310/europes-covid-19-hotspots-to-be-sent-million-four-million-more-vaccine-doses/> accessed 17 March 2021.

[18] 'EU toughens rules for vaccine exports to avoid shortfalls', The Local, 24 March 2021, <https://www.thelocal.se/20210324/eu-toughens-rules-for-vaccine-exports-to-avoid-shortfalls/> accessed 25 March 2021.

[19] 'Stockholm pushes back Covid-19 vaccine deadline', *The Local*, 15 February 2021, <https://www.thelocal.se/20210215/stockholm-pushes-back-covid-19-vaccine-deadline> and, 'Share of people vaccinated against COVID-19, February 14, 2021 & March 16, 2021' (Cumulative, and relative to population), and, 'Number of people fully vaccinated against COVID-19, February 14, 2021 & March 16, 2021,' Our World in Data, COVID-19 dataset, <https://ourworldindata.org> accessed 13 January 2022.

[20] Our World in Data, COVID-19 dataset, as note 19, March 31, April 30, May 31, June 30, and July 16.

[21] 'Sweden to introduce digital vaccine passport', *The Local*, 4 February 2021, <https://www.thelocal.se/20210204/sweden-to-introduce-vaccine-passport> accessed 17 February 2021.

[22] 'Could health passports kickstart travel around Europe', *The Local*, 18 March 2021, <https://www.thelocal.se/20210318/could-health-passports-kickstart-travel-around-europe/> accessed 21 March 2021.

[23] 'New COVID-19 variants now dominate in half of Sweden's regions', *The Local*, 16 March 2021, <https://www.thelocal.se/20210316/new-covid-19-variants-now-dominate-in-half-of-swedens-regions/> accessed 21 March 2021.

[24] 'Pressure on Sweden's healthcare increases as COVID-19 patients in ICUs rise to 292', *The Local*, 25 March 2021, <https://www.thelocal.se/20210325/pressure-on-swedens-healthcare-increases-as-covid-19-patients-in-icus-rise-to-292/> accessed 25 March 2021.

[25] Hancock, Sam. 'AstraZeneca vaccine: No evidence to restrict use of Covid jab, says EMA boss says', *The Independent*, 31 March 2021, <https://www.independent.co.uk/news/health/astrazeneca-oxford-covid-vaccine-ema-b1825082.html> accessed 1 April 2021.

[26] 'Explained: Why is Sweden waiting to restart AstraZeneca vaccinations?', *The Local*, 19 March 2021, <https://www.thelocal.se/20210319/explained-why-is-sweden-waiting-to-restart-astrazeneca-vaccinations/> accessed 21 March 2021.

[27] 'Vaccine acceptance could be lower after AstraZeneca pause, warns Swedish disease expert', *The Local*, 22 March 2021, <https://www.thelocal.se/20210322/vaccine-acceptance-could-be-lower-after-astrazeneac-pause-warns-swedish-disease-expert/> accessed 25 March 2021.

[28] Norberg, Johan. 'Sweden during the pandemic. Pariah or paragon?' p. 10, *CATO policy analysis*, No. 959, 29 August 2023, Cato Institute, <https://www.cato.org/sites/cato.org/files/2023-08/policy-analysis-959-no-link.pdf> accessed 6 February 2025.

[29] *The Local*, 22 March 2021, as note 27.

[30] Lichfield, John. 'Opinion: European governments were cautious on AstraZeneca vaccines but they were neither stupid nor political', *The Local*, 19 March 2021, <https://www.thelocal.se/20210319/opinion-european-governments-were-cautious-on-astrazeneca-vaccines-but-they-were-neither-stupid-nor-political/> accessed 22 March 2021.

[31] Ibid.

32 'AstraZeneca's Covid-19 vaccine: EMA finds possible link to very rare cases of unusual blood clots with low blood platelets', News, European Medicines Agency, 7 April 2021, <https://www.ema.europa.eu/en/news/astrazenecas-covid-19-vaccine-ema-finds-possible-link-very-rare-cases-unusual-blood-clots-low-blood> accessed 8 April 2021.

33 'Covid-19 third wave: Which countries in Europe have the tightest restrictions', *The Local*, 23 March 2021, <https://www.thelocal.se/20210323/covid-19-across-europe-how-countries-are-tightening-restrictions-while-others-are-easing-them/> accessed 25 March 2021.

34 Ibid.

35 Mackenzie, Jean. 'How Iceland clamped down to conquer coronavirus', *BBC News*, 23 March 2021, <https://www.bbc.co.uk/news/world-europe-56412790> accessed 24 March 2021.

36 Ibid.

37 Ibid.

38 'WHO-convened Global Study of Origins of SARS-CoV-2: China Part', Joint WHO- China Study 14 January-10 February 2021, Joint Report, WHO, Annex B, pp. 25–28, <https://www.who.int/docs/default-source/coronaviruse/who-convened-global-study-of-origins-of-sars-cov-2-china-part-annexes.pdf> accessed 31 March 2021.

39 'WHO-convened Global Study of Origins of SARS-CoV-2: China Part', Joint WHO- China Study 14 January-10 February 2021, Joint Report, WHO, pp. 7–8, <https://www.who.int/publications/i/item/who-convened-global-study-of-origins-of-sars-cov-2-china-part> accessed 30 March 2021.

40 Ibid., p. 8.

41 Ibid., p. 9.

42 Summary of the 'Final report: Covid select concludes 2-year investigation, issues 500+ page final report on lessons learned and the path forward', Press release, US Congress, House of Representatives, Committee on Oversight and Government Reform, 2 December 2024, <https://oversight.house.gov/release/final-report-covid-select-concludes-2-year-investigation-issues-500-page-final-report-on-lessons-learned-and-the-path-forward/> accessed 21 March 2025. The Select Subcommittee on the Coronavirus Pandemic, published 4 December 2024, was chaired by Brad Wenstrup.

43 'Covid-19 shows why united action is needed for more robust international health architecture', Commentary, WHO, 30 March 2021, <https://www.who.int/news-room/commentaries/detail/op-ed---covid-19-shows-why-united-action-is-needed-for-more-robust-international-health-architecture> accessed 1 April 2021.

44 Ibid.

45 Ibid.

46 'An international treaty on pandemic prevention and preparedness', European Council / Council of the European Union, 30 March 2021, <https://www.consilium.europa.eu/en/policies/coronavirus/pandemic-treaty/> accessed 1 April 2021.

47 Ibid.

48 'Sweden's response in the global fight against the COVID-19 pandemic', Ministry for Foreign Affairs, 19 March 2021, <https://www.government.se/articles/2021/03/swedens-response-in-the-global-fight-against-the-covid-19-virus/> accessed 2 April 2021.

49 Ibid.

50 'Carl Bildt, former prime Minister of Sweden, appointed WHO Special Envoy for the ACT-Accelerator', News release, WHO, 31 March 2021, <https://www.who.int/news/item/31-03-2021-carl-bildt-former-prime-minister-of-sweden-appointed-who-special-envoy-for-the-act-accelerator> accessed 2 April 2021.

51 Ibid.

Continuing Onslaught

Renewed Lockdowns – WHO Call to Ban Live Animal Sales in Food Markets

Into April 2021, Europe was still struggling with vaccine rollout, and Hans Kluge, WHO regional director, said that European programmes were 'unacceptably slow' and prolonging the pandemic in the region. To speed up the programmes, manufacturing of vaccines had to be ramped up, barriers to administering them had to be reduced, and every single vial had to be used – and now.[1]

The WHO had also given warning that the religious holidays of Pesach, Easter, and then Ramadan, that fell close together between end-March into April, would bring additional mobility and gatherings, and the risk of greater spread.[2]

Across the WHO Europe region, more than half of its fifty countries had implemented partial or full coronavirus lockdowns.[3] In Sweden, the public health agency called for a delay to the relaxations scheduled for April, particularly those for seated public events, indoors and outdoors. Planned relaxations ought to be held over until May, suggested the agency. Following on from that advice, Stefan Löfven, Lena Hallengren, and Johan Carlson, announced at a press conference that several of the coronavirus measures would be extended rather than relaxed. The spread of infection had to fall significantly, and pressure on the healthcare system had to be reduced, the prime minister said.

Although the WHO final report into the origins of COVID-19 had come to no firm conclusion about the role of the Huanan market in Wuhan, or how the infection was introduced into the market, officials believed that live animal markets posed a big risk in creating novel viruses in the future. So, in April, the WHO called for a complete ban on the sale of live animals in traditional food markets. To reduce public health risks, the organisation urged all governments to suspend the trade in live caught wild animals of mammalian species slaughtered and sold next to other foods.[4]

Continuing Anxiety Over Blood Clots – Oxford/AstraZeneca and EU Contract – Tegnell Takes His First Dose of Vaxzevria – Vaccination Among Elderly Migrants

Amid concerns about rare cases of blood clots, in mid-April Denmark became the first European country to cease giving Vaxzevria (the Oxford/AstraZeneca vaccine) in its vaccination programme. The decision would of course bring delay to the Danish programme, although the country had other vaccines available, and the virus was under control.[5]

For similar blood-clotting reasons – a rare risk – the USA, Canada, and the EU had paused use of the Johnson & Johnson (Janssen Pharmaceuticals) vaccine in April. South Africa too had paused its use despite the vaccine being the preferred one in the fight against the Beta-variant of COVID-19.[6] In Europe, delay to the rollout of the Johnson & Johnson vaccine would impact the vaccination programmes of several countries. The rollout had been on hold in Sweden, which had been expecting to receive 1.2 million doses alongside its Pfizer BioNTech, Vaxzevria, and Moderna vaccines.

Because of shortfalls in deliveries of Vaxzevria by AstraZeneca, it was beginning to look likely that the EU would not renew contracts with the UK-Swedish company. Thierry Breton, the EU commissioner responsible for vaccine supply said that AstraZeneca had committed to supply 120 million doses to the EU in the first quarter of 2021, but had delivered only 30 million, and had cut the second quarter commitment from 180 million to 70 million doses. Contracts were due to expire at the end of June. Von der Leyen announced that in the second quarter the EU would receive an extra 50 million doses of the Pfizer/BioNTech vaccine to partly make up for the Vaxzevria shortfall. The EU Commission was also in talks with Pfizer/BioNTech for 1.8 billion doses in 2022 and 2023. The company had 'delivered on its commitments' and was 'responsive to our needs', von der Leyen said. The EU needed to focus on technologies that had 'proven their worth', and Pfizer/BioNTech had 'proven to be a reliable partner'.[7] It was not looking good for AstraZeneca.

Meanwhile, in Sweden, and himself recently having become 65-years old, Tegnell had been vaccinated with a first dose of Vaxzevria at a vaccination hub in Linköping. Amid reports that people were refusing Vaxzevria, he had wanted to send an important signal that it was a great vaccine for the over-65s. In publicity around the 'event', he said that it had also been important to know how large the problem of refusal was, and what information was needed to help people make the right choices. The vaccine had to be used to the maximum, and to reach as many people as possible, as quickly as possible, he had added.[8] It had been reported that in some Swedish regions, doses were having to be thrown away.

Not being reached were elderly foreign-born residents and there was concern across the country about that. Indeed, among immigrants to Sweden generally, there was a worryingly low vaccination rate. Of those people over-80 who had been born in sub-Saharan Africa, only 44 per cent had been vaccinated, of those born in North Africa 59 per cent had been vaccinated, and of those born in the EU and North America 77 per cent and 81 per cent respectively had been vaccinated. This compared to the 85 per cent vaccination rate of those over-80 born in the other Nordic countries, and the 91 per cent of those born in Sweden.[9]

Tegnell said that the differences in vaccination uptake were worrying for several reason, but not least because the elderly in any group had been the hardest hit, and in the long run 'uneven vaccine cover' risked new outbreaks and renewed social spread. The vaccination programme would need new measures and targeted efforts to reach the elderly foreign-born. About 20 per cent of the population of Sweden had been born in another country (19.7 per cent in 2020, and 20 per cent in 2021), and studies had shown that there was higher risk of serious illness from COVID-19 among people with lower education, lower income, and among those living in overcrowded conditions. Immigrant groups were very heterogeneous, so a mix of outreach would have to be made.[10]

Rising Infection Rates – Eurovision 2021 – Vaccination Milestone – 'Green Digital Certificates'

Into April, the rate of infection had reached the level of the previous peak, and several Swedish regions had reached maximum capacity for intensive care and had been forced to seek assistance from other areas. Region Västernorrland, Region Kalmar County, and Region Örebro had seen particularly high levels of infection, along with the city regions around Stockholm, Gothenburg and Malmö.

The rising infection rate brought renewed calls from the public health agency for people to be aware of their behaviour. There would be no easing of restrictions until pressure on healthcare had decreased and the spread of infection had gone down. Indeed, some municipalities banned gatherings in public parks for Valborg 2021 revelries – the second year running that *Valborgsmässoafton* or *Walpurgisnacht* had been curtailed. In May though, across in the Netherlands, in front of an audience all having tested negative to COVID-19, the Eurovision Song Contest did take place, in Rotterdam, the scheduled city for the cancelled 2020 event, with Sweden represented this time by Tusse (Tussaint Michael Chiza), a Congolese-Swede.

Closely following the EU proposal for digital certification providing information about vaccination status, and going under the name '*gröna beviset*', Sweden's 'green digital certificate' or vaccine pass was unveiled in April. The digital certificate would be free of charge and contain a QR code (Quick Response code, a type of barcode) with information about the vaccine received, and when, along with personal information. Analogue certification was also being worked on, to allow everyone the same opportunity, to travel, say, but it was likely to take a little longer to find a solution. It would also be possible to save the digital vaccination certificate and to print it out, and perhaps to apply for it digitally but receive it in the post.[11]

A prerequisite for the system to work properly was correct reporting across the regions into the national vaccination register (*Vaccinationsregistret*, at the Public Health Agency). This would perhaps be a tough ask when the healthcare system was under such pressure, but it was essential for subsequent issue of the certificate. While the EU aimed to allow vaccination certificates to be used from 26 June, in Sweden those seeking them would be able to visit the Swedish eHealth agency website (*eHälsomyndigheten*) from 1 July, and within seven days of vaccination and its reporting by healthcare staff to the national register.[12]

Although the purpose of certification was to facilitate travel within the EU, not least for those commuting across national borders – between Malmö and Copenhagen and crossing Øresundsbron (the Öresund Bridge), for example – it would still be up to individual member states to decide on what would be required to enter their countries. For most Swedes, it would probably be mainly about holiday travel, but of course that was likely to need some planning, such as: getting the vaccination; the waiting time for the certificate; and, the destination, its travel requirements, and whether the certificate would be valid there.[13]

Later, the EU digital certificate came to be known as the EU Digital COVID Certificate, and after provisional agreement on the Commission proposal was reached between the European Parliament and the European Council on 20 May, it was set to come into force on 1 July 2021. Von der Leyen had welcomed the swift progress made on certification, saying that the commitment to have the EU Digital COVID Certificate up and running before the summer had been delivered on. It would free of charge, secure, accessible to all in paper or digital format, and cover vaccination, testing, and recovery. It would offer different options and fully respected fundamental rights including protection of personal data.[14] There would be no tangible product given out from Brussels – the EU Digital COVID Certificate was more of an agreement – and it would be the task of individual member states to develop their own digital solutions.

While the digital certificate enabled the fundamental right of EU citizens to free movement across the EU in the age of coronavirus, and to make it easier for Europeans to travel, it could also be used by member states for national purposes, if provided for in national law. Member states however were to refrain from imposing additional restrictions on holders of the certificate unless they were necessary and proportionate to the safeguarding of public health.[15]

The EU Digital COVID Certificate would also be used by Iceland, Liechtenstein, Norway, and Sweden.

On 1 July, the Swedish vaccine pass was launched as planned.

Continuing Onslaught of COVID-19 – India

In early-April, the global death toll from COVID-19 had passed 3,000,000 (milestone recorded 8 April 2021), and in the last week of the month there had been 1,000,000 deaths in Europe (recorded 25 April 2021).[16]

In India, a new wave of infection had brought the vast country the largest number of daily infections in the world. From 25 April, over 350,000 cases daily were being reported, well above the peak of 97,000 recorded in September 2020, and new peaks in late-April and early-May 2021 when India became the first country to record 400,000 new cases per day. In February 2021, daily cases had been as low as 9,000, with just over 135 daily deaths, while on 25 April over 2,800 deaths were recorded.[17]

Throughout the country, hospitals had run out of oxygen and ventilators as hospitals and ICUs had become overwhelmed by desperately ill people, and many of the scenes shown on television – frantic relatives searching for oxygen, desperate medical staff, makeshift funeral pyres – seemed post-apocalyptic. The new wave in India was still weeks away from peaking.

While the older Alpha-variant and a new Delta-variant (first identified in India itself) had been circulating since 2020, and lockdown had been in place since March, the damaging wave of cases could have been caused by large gatherings – religious festivals and election rallies – and a lack of preventive measures such as face-coverings and social distancing.[18] Complacency had also been a factor.

While the outbreak in India had been serious, the size of the country and its population of 1.38 billion 'hid' the country in global COVID-19 statistics. On 25 April, as far as cumulative confirmed COVID-19 deaths per million people were concerned, India had recorded 141.03 deaths while dozens of other countries throughout the world had suffered far more on the same measure. For the sake of comparison, out of these dozens of countries, Paraguay had recorded 817.22, South Africa 901.84, Europe 1,335.49, Chile 1,345.8, Sweden 1,370.35, EU 1,514.26, France 1,525.79, Mexico 1,650.11, Brazil 1,827.92, the UK 1,869.51, Italy 1,975.2, Czechia 2,700.53, and Hungary had recorded 2,763.6.[19] Norway with a population of 5.5 million was only slightly 'better' than India on this measure with 134.66 cumulative deaths per million.

On 16 July 2020, India and Sweden had come close to recording similar daily new confirmed COVID-19 cases per million people, with Sweden recording 26.87 cases per million people, and India recording 25.1. Again, on 25 September

2020, the two countries had come close, with Sweden recording 62.4 cases per million people, and India recording 61.26.

Statistics could always paint a different picture from the reality on the ground, and in spring 2021, India had found itself overwhelmed by the coronavirus. Barely one tenth of the vast population had been vaccinated, and yet the country had been the largest exporter of COVID-19 vaccines to the rest of the world. So that it would have enough doses to fully vaccinate its own population by November 2021, the Indian government brought in a temporary ban on the export of vaccines. This would of course lead to shortages elsewhere, particularly lower-income countries. Indeed, India was to have produced more than 80 per cent of the 2.26 billion doses to the COVAX initiative.[20]

By 6 May, India had recorded 21.49 million cumulative confirmed cases of COVID-19, and 234,083 cumulative confirmed deaths. A month later, on 6 June, confirmed cases had risen to 28.91 million, and deaths had risen to 349,186.[21]

In a further comparison, in Brazil on 6 June, cumulative confirmed cases had reached 16.95 million, and there had been 473,741 deaths. Over the 24-hour period between 18 and 19 June, Brazil had recorded 500,000 deaths. On the measure of cumulative confirmed COVID-19 deaths per million people, India had suffered 277.53 on 19 June, and Brazil 2,341.7.[22]

1,000,000 Cumulative Confirmed Cases in Sweden – May Day Protests

By 6 May too, Sweden had passed another milestone statistic, having recorded 1 million cumulative confirmed cases since the start of the pandemic.[23] The actual number was likely to have been much larger, of course, with many potential cases going untested and the asymptomatic shedding the virus to others.

That approaching milestone had not been enough to sway many from gathering over May Day despite the rules against mass gatherings. Protest against coronavirus restrictions brought hundreds to a square in Stockholm – Norra Bantorget – which in turn led to police intervention to disperse the crowd. When ordered to leave, the crowd ignored the police and carried on in a march towards Odenplan (another central city square) and then to Vasaparken (a city park). There had been a couple of instances of 'violent resistance' and a police vehicle was attacked. At the park, speakers argued that the 'digital certificates' or 'vaccine passes' (otherwise known as EU Digital COVID Certificates), were a form of 'medical apartheid'. During the event, chants of 'Wake up Sweden' were shouted, and some signs carried messages of 'COVID-19 was planned', and 'Mass media is the virus'. Organisers of the march, which had been called the '1st May Protest for Freedom and Truth' (or *Majtåget för Frihet och Sanning*) were issued with fines of SEK 3,000 each, and one person had been arrested.[24]

A similar protest had taken place in Stockholm earlier in the spring, in March – at Medborgarplatsen – and a common feature of the gatherings, in addition to protest against coronavirus restrictions and the Pandemic Law, had been claims about 5G health risks, claims against vaccines (anti-vaxxers), and general conspiracy theories. Some believed that vaccination was part of a conspiracy led by powerful people in the pharmaceutical industry and elsewhere.[25]

There would be no early relaxing of restrictions in Sweden, however. The spread of infection in the country was among the highest in the EU, and the health system was still being stretched. An easing of restrictions was unlikely before June.

Vaccination Across Europe

After a sluggish start, the pace of vaccination across Europe had picked up markedly into May 2021.

In Germany, a daily 1.1 million doses were being given, and in France 500,000 daily, and Spain 300,000. In the EU, Denmark was leading on the measure of share of population fully vaccinated, due to its decision to keep a short 3-week gap between the first and second doses in its Pfizer/BioNTech and Moderna vaccination programmes (extended to a 6-week gap in April). By 11 May, nearly 16 per cent of Danes had been fully vaccinated (all doses), with Spain, Switzerland, Italy, and France not far behind. In Iceland just over 15 per cent of the population had been fully vaccinated, in Norway nearly 10 per cent, in Sweden just over 9 per cent, and in Finland nearly 4 per cent. In the UK it was just over 27 per cent.[26]

On 13 May, over 1 million people in Sweden had been fully vaccinated (1.07 million).

Reopening of Sweden – Ongoing Vaccination Programme

At the beginning of June, a five-step re-opening plan got underway in Sweden.

It would see a second step on 1 July, a third in mid-July, a fourth in September, and then a fifth lifting all remaining rules and recommendations at an indeterminate date (each step being decided by the epidemiological situation). The plan would define the relaxation of rules and recommendations relevant to events and gatherings, eating and drinking, face-coverings, and travel.[27]

On 1 June, the cap was raised on numbers attending public events, allowing up to fifty people in cinemas, theatres, and other seated indoor events, up to 100 at non-seated sports, cultural, and other outdoor events, up to 500 at seated sports, cultural, and other outdoor events, and up to 150 people at running, orienteering, swimming, and other outdoor competitive events. At events such as flea markets, and at permanent amusement parks like Liseberg (in Gothenburg), Gröna Lund (Stockholm), and Skara Sommarland (Scandinavia's largest, situated in Västra Götaland), people would be allowed to circulate at one person per 20 sq m. Bars and restaurants would be able to remain open until 22.30 with a maximum of four per table, and with table service only. Masks and other face-coverings were still recommended on public transport during rush hour, but in some regions of Sweden it was advised at all times, as well as in confined indoor spaces such as shops, pharmacies, hairdressers, as well as visits to dentist, doctor, and hospital.[28]

Returning to the workplace would not be part of the first phase of the reopening plan. The recommendation from the public health agency was to continue working from home as far as possible. This recommendation, along with staying at home if anyone experienced COVID-19 symptoms, keeping a distance from others, limiting contacts by socializing only with a social bubble, and avoiding any environment where there was a risk of crowding, were expected to remain in place until autumn 2021.[29]

From 1 July, restaurants and bars were able to open until 02.00 (pre-pandemic hours), and for outdoor seating caps on the number of customers sitting together had been removed. Indoors, tables had to be a metre apart. Measures to curb the spread of infection stayed in place – keeping distance at checkouts and providing the necessary hand-washing opportunity. At seated indoor events 300 people were allowed, and 3,000 at outdoor events. For events without designated seating, a cap was set at 50 people indoors, 600 outdoors, and 900 at running events and other competitive events. Up to 1,800 people could gather at an outdoor demonstration. In shops, gyms, and other similar businesses, people would be allowed to circulate at one person per 10 sq m of usable space. On public transport, the national recommendation on wearing face-coverings was lifted, though these still applied in some regions. Buses and trains travelling distances over 150 km. could only run at half capacity. The advice on working from home remained in place, but the national recommendation to only meet people in one's immediate circle was lifted and replaced with the advice to meet outdoors and in small groups away from others in restricted spaces.[30]

Critical to the reopening of the country was the ongoing vaccination programme, and into June it appeared that vaccination rates among the older foreign-born population had risen after concerns earlier in the year. According to the public health agency, during the three weeks up to mid-June the vaccination rate among those born outside Sweden and aged 60–64 had risen from 59 per cent to 67 per cent. Even so, coverage remained lower than that for people born in Sweden in the same age group and over the same period which had seen a rise from 83 per cent to 88 per cent. Hitherto, the lowest rate of vaccination had been among people born in the sub-region south of the North African countries. Nevertheless, over the same period vaccine coverage had jumped from 49 per cent to 61 per cent.[31]

Into June too, vaccination booking had opened to anyone over the age of thirty-five and to those born in 1986 who had not yet had their birthday in 2021. Those who had been eligible in earlier vaccination phases and risk groups but who had not yet received a vaccine were also still able to get one. Those in the 30–34 age group would be able to get vaccinations later in June or in July, and by August the 18–29 age group would be eligible.[32] While this reflected vaccination progress in Stockholm, there would be regional differences across the country.

Back in December 2020, Hallengren had said that by 26 June 2021 all eligible adults would have been offered their first dose of a COVID-19 vaccine. However, the reality was that just ahead of the Midsummer weekend and the start of Sweden's long summer closedown the share of the adult population having at least one dose of vaccine was 45.66 per cent. Delays in vaccine deliveries had been to blame, and the target of having all adults offered their first dose had been put back to 19 September at the latest.[33]

By end-June, five of Sweden's regions had opened vaccination bookings for all over-18s, with Region Västra Götaland joining Region Norrbotten, Region Jönköping, Region Södermanland (Sörmland), and Region Västernorrland, a month ahead of schedule. During early-July, Region Halland and Region Örebro had opened to over-18s too. In Region Stockholm and Region Skåne, vaccinations had become available to more young adults – those in their 20s.[34] More and more Swedish regions would open bookings for all over-18s, and by mid-July when Region Uppsala made them available, every region had done so.

By mid-July, the share of the Swedish population fully vaccinated against COVID-19, with first and second doses, was 38 per cent, or 3.86 million. Those having at least one dose of COVID-19 vaccine was 21.78 per cent, or 2.21 million.[35] Although statistics had shown that more and more people were fully vaccinated, this did not mean that those having only one of the protocol doses had lessened in step with that. The previously unvaccinated may have stepped forward for their first dose, and older teenagers now counted as adults would also form part of a new mix or set.

Into August, and after a recommendation from the public health agency, several regions were planning to open vaccination bookings to the over-16s, and some had already done so, though September looked more likely for other regions.[36]

Statistics, July 2021 – Delta-Variant in Sweden – Coronavirus Cases in Decline Overall – World Deaths – Delta-Variant in China

In mid-June, the public health agency stated for the first time that there had been a spread of the Delta-variant of coronavirus in several Swedish regions, though it was too early to say if the variant would become dominant.

At a national level, no major adaptation of the country's COVID-19 measures had been introduced to meet the spread, though there had been an increase in the proportion of test results being sequenced to identify variants. At a regional and local level where an outbreak had occurred, sometimes a school or a nursery, a shop, or maybe a football club might be closed, and sporting tournaments and matches cancelled.[37] The spread of the Delta-variant had not been expected to delay Sweden's reopening plan however, and relaxations planned for 1 July went ahead.

In early-July though, the public health agency said that the more contagious variant was likely to become the dominant one in Sweden before autumn, and advised cautious behaviour, particularly as regards the number of people mixed with. Nevertheless, cases of COVID-19 overall were in decline. As of 1 July, the country's incidence rate had fallen to 55.41 daily new cases per million, less than the EU at 56.39, and much less than Europe over all at 105.09. In Denmark the incidence rate was 81.71, in Finland 40.01, Norway 35.31, and Iceland there had been none. In the UK, the rate had been 404.96. On 1 April, Sweden had recorded 817.41 daily new cases per million. In early-May, daily new cases had jumped up to 1,471.43 (4 May), and in early-June back down to 838.57 (3 June).[38]

On 6 July, the world reached a milestone of 4 million deaths. Of these, 1.11 million had occurred in Europe, 1.02 million in South America with more than half of them in Brazil, 905,290 in North America with two thirds of that figure in the USA, 809,186 in Asia with around half in India, 147,872 in Africa with South Africa and Nigeria accounting for around half, and 910 in Australia.[39]

By mid-July, the Delta-variant had made up 60 per cent of new COVID-19 cases in Sweden, and the Alpha-variant 30 per cent.[40] The Delta-variant was now the dominant one in the country, just as the public health agency said it would become.

In early-August, there had been concerns in China about outbreaks of the Delta-variant across fifteen provinces, with many connected to an outbreak that began in Nanjing in eastern Jiangsu. These cases had been traced back to an outbreak among airport workers in Nanjing who had cleaned a plane that had arrived from Russia. In the city, 9.2 million people were tested, and a lockdown imposed. In Zhuzhou, in central Hunan province, over a million people were told to stay at home while mass testing and mass-vaccinations were carried out. The Delta-variant had also reached Wuhan in Hubei province from where COVID-19 had first been reported to the world back in December 2019. The spread throughout China had been attributed to the domestic summer tourist season. Transport links between Beijing and areas with positive cases had been cut, and tourists were banned from entering the city.[41]

Chapter 9 examines life alongside COVID-19 in the period August to December 2021, particularly new spread and spikes, and new border closures and travel bans. It describes efforts by Øresundsbron (the Øresund Bridge) to kickstart cross-border connections again and to encourage cross-border job-seeking, and the restarting of Norway–Sweden rail services. It examines the differing guidance for the vaccinated and unvaccinated, and how, towards the end of the year, Sweden was among those countries showing the lowest infection spread in Europe. Finally, it looks at the emergence of the Omicron-variant and its effects.

Notes

1 'Covid: Europe's vaccine rollout unacceptably slow - WHO', *BBC News*, 1 April 2021, <https://www.bbc.co.uk/news/world-europe-56600660> accessed 2 April 2021.

2 Ibid.

3 Ibid.

4 Forrest, Adam. 'WHO calls for ban on sale of live animals in food markets to combat pandemics', *The Independent*, 13 April 2021, <https://www.independent.co.uk/news/health/covid-live-animals-markets-ban-b1830469.html> accessed 25 April 2021.

5 'AstraZeneca vaccine: Denmark stops rollout completely', *BBC News*, 14 April 2021, <https://www.bbc.co.uk/news/world-europe-56744474> accessed 25 April 2021.

6 Ibid.

7 Henley, Jon. 'EU may not renew vaccine contract with AstraZeneca over delivery shortfalls', *The Guardian*, 19 April 2021, <https://www.guardian.com/world/live/2021/apr/19/coronavirus-live-news-uk-study-to-expose-young-people-to-virus-for-second-time-india-cases-top-15m?page=with:block-607d864c8f08080a7ae65457> accessed 25 April 2021.

8 Holmgren Mia. 'Tegnell: Största utmaningen är att nå ut med relevant information om Astras vaccin', *Dagens Nyheter*, 20 April 2021, <https://www.dn.se/sverige/tegnell-storsta-utmaningen-ar-att-na-ut-med-relevant-information-om-astras-vaccin/> and, 'Sweden's state epidemiologist Anders Tegnell gets Astra Zeneca vaccine', *The Local*, 19 April 2021, <https://thelocal.se/20210419/swedens-state-epidemiologist-anders-tegnell-gets-astra-zeneca-covid-vaccine> accessed 21 April 2021.

9 Tanaka, Sofia. and Gustav Olsson. 'Lägre andel bland utlandsfödda som vaccinerar sig', *Dagens Nyheter*, 29 April 2021, <https://www.dn.se/sverige/lagre-andel-bland-utlandsfodda-som-vaccinerar-sig/> accessed 30 April.

10 Ibid., and SCB Table 'Population of Sweden by country/region of birth, citizenship and Swedish/foreign background, 31 December 202 and 2021', *Statistikmyndigheten SCB*. The table showed that for both years, those born in Syria showed the highest percentage among Sweden's foreign-born, at 1.9 per cent in both 2020 and 2021. Those born in Iraq

showed 1.4 per cent both years, and those born in Finland showed 1.3 per cent in 2020 and 1.4 per cent in 2021. Somalis accounted for 0.7 per cent in both years.

11 'Gröna beviset kan öppna för resor', *Dagens Nyheter*, 26 April 2021, <https://www.dn.se/varlden/grona-beviset-kan-oppna-for-resor/> accessed 29 April 2021.

12 Ibid., and 'How to get your vaccine pass in Sweden', *The Local*, 11 June 2021, <https://www.thelocal.se/20210611/how-to-get-your-covid-19-vaccine-pass-in-sweden/> accessed 20 June 2021. E-health concerned digital tools and sharing information digitally to achieve and maintain good levels of health, and included e-prescriptions, electronic medical records, and appointments booked online.

13 *Dagens Nyheter*, 26 April 2021, as note 11.

14 'EU Digital COVID Certificate: European Parliament and Council reach agreement on Commission proposal', European Commission, Press release, 20 May 2021, <https://ec.europa.eu/commission/presscorner/detail/en/ip_21_2593> accessed 24 May 2021.

15 Ibid.

16 'Cumulative confirmed COVID-19 deaths, April 8 and April 25, 2021, Our World in Data, COVID-19 dataset, <https://ourworldindata.org> accessed 13 January 2022.

17 'Daily new confirmed COVID-19 deaths, April 25, 2021, Our World in Data, COVID- 19 dataset, <https://ourworldindata.org> accessed 13 January 2022.

18 Biswas, Soutik. 'What is the Indian COVID variant and will vaccines work?' *BBC News*, 23 April 2021, <https://www.bbc.co.uk/news/world-asia-india-56844925> accessed 26 April 2021.

19 'Cumulative COVID-19 deaths per million people, April 25, 2021', Our World in Data, COVID-19 dataset, <https://ourworldindata.org> accessed 13 January 2022.

20 Garcia, Carmen Aguilar. and Ganesh Rao. 'Covid-19: India's vaccine export ban could send shockwaves worldwide. Should the UK step in to help?', Sky News, 30 April 2021, <https://news.sky.com/story/covid-19-how-does-indias-pause-on-vaccine-export-hurt-other-nations-12290300> accessed 13 May 2021.

21 'Cumulative confirmed COVID-19 deaths per million people, May 6, and June 6, 2021', and 'Cumulative confirmed COVID-19 cases, May 6, and June 6, 2021', Our World in Data, COVID-19 dataset, <https://ourworldindata.org> accessed 14 January 2022.

22 'Cumulative confirmed COVID-19 cases, June 6, 2021', and 'Cumulative confirmed COVID-19 deaths per million people, June 19, 2021', and 'Cumulative confirmed COVID-19 deaths per million people, June 6, 2021', Our World in Data, COVID-19 dataset, <https://ourworldindata.org> accessed 14 January 2022.

23 'Cumulative confirmed COVID-19 cases, May 6, 2021', Our World in Data, COVID-19 dataset, <https://ourworldindata.org> accessed 14 January 2022.

24 Carp, Ossi. and Amanda Lindholm, Alexandra Carlsson Tenitskaja. 'En gripen och ett tiotal brottsmisstänkta efter anti-coronademonstration i Stockholm', *Dagens Nyheter*, 1 May 2021, <https://www.dn.se/sthlm/polisen-upploser-coronademonstration-i-stockholm/> and, 'Police take two hours to disperse Stockholm anti-lockdown protest', *The Local*, 2 May 2021, <https://www.thelocal.se/20210502/police-take-two-hours-to-disperse-stockholm-anti-lockdown-protest/> accessed 13 May 2021.

25 Carp and Lindholm, *Dagens Nyheter*, as note 24.

26 'Share of the population fully vaccinated against COVID-19, May 11, 2021, Our World in Data, COVID-19 dataset, <https://ourworldindata.org> accessed 14 January 2022.

27 'Six essential articles to help you navigate Sweden's pandemic reopening plan', *The Local*, 1 June 2021, <https://www.thelocal.se/20210601/six-handy-articles-to-help-you-navigate-swedens-reopening-plan/> accessed 3 June 2021.

28 Ibid.

[29] 'Work from home until at least end of September: Swedish Public Health Agency', *The Local*, 16 June 2021, <https://www.thelocal.se/20210616/work-from-home-until-at-least-end-of-september-swedish-public-health-agency/> accessed 21 June 2021.

[30] 'What Covid-19 rules and restrictions apply in Sweden now?', *The Local*, 1 July 2021, <https://www.thelocal.se/20210701/what-covid-19-rules-and-restrictions-apply-in-sweden-now-july-2021/> accessed 3 July 2021.

[31] 'New stats: Vaccination rate rises among foreign-born people in Sweden', *The Local*, 14 June 2021, <https://www.thelocal.se/20210614/vaccination-rate-rises-among-foreign-born-people-in-sweden/> accessed 20 June 2021.

[32] 'Stockholm opens vaccinations to over 35s – here's how to book your Covid shot', *The Local*, 11 May 2021, updated 14 June 2021, <https://www.thelocal.se/20210511/how-do-i-book-my-covid-19-vaccination-in-stockholm/> accessed 20 June 2021.

[33] 'COVID-19 vaccine doses, people with at least one dose, people fully vaccinated, and boosters per 100 people, June 21, 2021', Our World in Data, COVID-19 dataset, <https://ourworldindata.org> accessed 14 January 2022, and, 'Sweden postpones its Covid-19 vaccine target again', *The Local*, 24 June 2021, <https://www.thelocal.se/20210624/sweden-postpones-its-covid-19-vaccine-target-again/> accessed 2 July 2021.

[34] Milford, Chiara. 'Five of Sweden's regions open COVID-19 vaccine booking to all over-18s', *The Local*, 30 June 2021, <https://www.thelocal.se/20210630/five-of-swedens-regions-open-covid-19-vaccine-booking-to-all-over-18s/> accessed 3 July 2021.

[35] 'Share of vaccinated against COVID-19, July 16, 2021' & 'Number of people vaccinated against COVID-19, July 16, 2021', Our World in Data, COVID-19 dataset, <https://ourworldindata.org> accessed 14 January 2022.

[36] 'Explained: What changes about life in Sweden in August 2021?' *The Local*, 2 August 2021, <https://www.thelocal.se/20210726/explained-what-changes-about-life-in-sweden-in-august-2021/> accessed 2 August 2021.

[37] Edwards, Catherine. 'How concerned should we be about the spread of the Delta COVID-19 variant in Sweden?', *The Local*, 17 June 2021, <https://www.thelocal.se/20210617/how-concerned-should-we-be-about-the-spread-of-the-delta-covid-19-variant-in-sweden/> accessed 2 July 2021.

[38] 'Daily new confirmed COVID-19 cases per million people, July 1, 2021', and April 1, May 4, and June 3, Our World in Data, COVID-19 dataset, <https://ourworldindata.org> accessed 14 January 2022.

[39] 'Cumulative confirmed COVID-19 deaths, July 6, 2021', Our World in Data, COVID -19 dataset, <https://ourworldindata.org> accessed 14 January 2022.

[40] 'Delta variant now makes up 60 per cent of new COVID cases in Sweden', *The Local*, 16 July 2021, <https://www.thelocal.se/20210716/delta-variant-now-makes-up-60-per-cent-of-new-covid-cases-in-sweden/> accessed 17 July 2021.

[41] 'Nanjing: Concerns in China grow as Delta outbreak spreads', *BBC News*, 2 August 2021, <https://www.bbc.co.uk/news/world-asia-china-58052894> accessed 3 August 2021.

Renewing Connexions

Spread and Spike – Schools – Border Closure – Violating EU Rules – Travel Bans and Exemptions

Well into August 2021, as Sweden began to waken up from the traditional long summer shutdown, the public health agency indicated that new coronavirus cases were on the rise and that people should continue to follow the recommendations to stem the spread of the virus. While the number of cases had increased, the number of new deaths was still very low.[1] So far it was a question of cases, not consequences.

People were being urged to continue working from home where possible. This recommendation was to remain in place until end-September and could be extended. Separately, prime minister Stefan Löfven said at a press conference that the government would ask parliament to extend the temporary Pandemic Law until January 2022, and to extend temporary infection control measures in restaurants.[2]

At the same time, Sweden's professional association of teachers – *Lärarnas Riksförbund, LR* – had called on health authorities to let children over 12 be vaccinated against COVID-19. Currently it was being offered to over-16s. The association, in effect the national union of teachers, had said that with the increased spread of infection in society, it would be difficult, if not impossible, for schools to follow public health agency regulations to maintain distance among children.[3] Indeed, for Swedish schools which were set to announce the removal of preventive distance learning and a return to in-school teaching, public health agency instructions had been described as nonchalant and lacking systematic protection for children. While the agency had stuck to its view that children 'don't get sick from COVID-19', they could spread it to vulnerable family members and suffer post-COVID symptoms themselves and develop debilitating 'long-COVID' just like adults.[4]

After a spike of infection following the 'Tantra Week' festival in Molkom, just north of Karlstad in Värmland, in August, neighbouring Norway classified the Swedish province as a 'red region'. This meant that unvaccinated Swedes would be denied entry to Norway and those who had the right of entry had to be able to show a negative test as well as being tested at the border and be quarantined.[5]

Although the EU Digital COVID Certificate scheme had come into force on 1 July, it was obvious into August that Sweden was failing to offer the pass to everyone who was entitled to one. EU citizens living in Sweden without a Swedish social security number (a personal identity number, or *personnummer*) had been unable to order the official vaccine certificate. Despite EU rules stating that vaccinated people had the right to get the certificate from the member state administering their vaccine (EU regulation 2021/935, 14 June 2021), many were having to pay for a negative test to be able to travel freely – a violation of freedom of movement.[6]

Because COVID passes were issued on the basis of information obtained from the national vaccination centre – a system that required an individual to have a Swedish social security number – the government instructed the eHealth Agency to investigate how a manual routine for issuing COVID passes could be developed and implemented for those who had been vaccinated but for various reasons did not have a *personnummer*. A manual system would also enable those Swedes who had been vaccinated in third countries and who had moved back to Sweden, or who were staying for a longer time before going back, to obtain a COVID pass. The eHealth agency had until 1 October to report back, but when it did there appeared to be no easy solutions.[7] Nevertheless, the government insisted that these services had to be in place by the end of the year.[8]

Also in August, a ban in place since March 2020 on travel to Sweden from non-EU/EEA countries had been extended until 31 October. It had been expected to expire at end-August. This meant that a foreign citizen travelling to Sweden and departing from a state other than an EEA state or Switzerland would be denied entry and turned away. There were several exemptions from the ban, but even if covered by one of these exemptions travellers would still be required to present a negative COVID-19 test result. From 11 October, travellers who could present a vaccination certificate issued in the UK, for example, would be exempt from the ban on entry to Sweden and test requirement. The UK, by contrast, had allowed entry to fully vaccinated Swedes for some time.[9] Since late-September, citizens from several other countries had been exempted from the entry ban and requirement to present a negative test result – simply producing a vaccination certificate instead – and these were: Albania, Andorra, the Faroe Islands, Israel, Morocco, Monaco, and Panama.

In September it was announced that from 1 October the Swedish foreign ministry would lift its global travel advisory, meaning that there would no longer be a recommendation against unnecessary travel from Sweden.

Øresundsbron Kickstarts Cross-Border Integration – Cross-Border Job Quests – Oslo-Gothenburg Rail Service to Restart

Following eighteen-months of disruption due to the pandemic and to encourage renewed travel between Sweden and Denmark, the Øresund Bridge consortium (Øresundsbron) announced the launch of a three-month discount offer to kick-start use of the bridge again.[10]

The Öresund Region – composed of Sweden's third city of Malmö and the Danish capital of Copenhagen and their regional hinterlands – was supposed to be a common metropolitan area but it had undergone division during the pandemic. The hospitality industry had been especially hard-hit. The number of overnight stays on either side of the Sound (the Öresund, a strait between Sweden and Denmark) had crashed to a record low during the first half of 2021. In Region Skåne, overnight stays in guest or tourist accommodation had decreased by 81 per cent compared with the first half of 2019. In the Capital Region of Denmark and Region Zealand, overnight stays of guests and tourists from Sweden had decreased by 91 per cent.[11]

The launch of a 'Buy one journey, Get one free' offer available between 1 September and 30 November 2021 was an attempt by the bridge consortium to inject greater optimism and to encourage increased travel on both sides of the Sound. Travellers using the bridge were offered favourable discounts in hotels across the Öresund Region. It was recognized too that more than one offer might be required to bring restart to the region, and different ways would have to found by business generally, the hospitality industry in particular, and politicians, to achieve this, and to restore confidence on either side of the bridge.[12]

Cross-border cooperation to match Danish jobs to Swedish jobseeker, and vice versa, had also gotten underway again by the autumn. One initiative was a collaboration between the Capital Region of Denmark, Malmö and Copenhagen municipalities, the Danish Chamber of Commerce (Dansk Ehrverv), and the Swedish Public Employment Service, aimed at solving a post-pandemic labour crisis on both sides of the Öresund and to fill 53,500 Danish private sector vacancies with 65,000 unemployed people in Region Skåne. The hotel and restaurant industries of the cross-border region had been struggling to fill vacancies, with several hotels keeping rooms closed because they had not been able to find staff.

The public employment service in Sweden had almost 124,000 jobs advertised on its site in September, which was up from the 60,000 advertised in September 2020, and 80,000 in September 2019.[13]

On the question of cross-border links between Norway and Sweden, the rail service between Oslo and Gothenburg which had been closed for eighteen-months because of the pandemic was set to start up again too. Although borders had begun to slowly open between Norway and Sweden, the rail service had remained closed due to difficulties in checking the test and vaccination status of passengers. To avoid confusion, all passengers would now be required to have a COVID certificate to board the train.[14]

Also set to resume was the Stockholm-Oslo rail service which would begin operating in December 2021. It would be operated at the same level as before the pandemic – two services per day.[15]

Inquiry Into Constitutional Preparedness for Future Pandemics – Appointed

In September 2021, the Swedish government appointed a commission of inquiry with the task of reviewing the Communicable Diseases Control Act and updating the legislation.

Lena Hallengren, the health and social affairs minister, said that by appointing the inquiry, advantage could be taken from the experience of COVID-19 to help and strengthen society's ability to better face future epidemics or pandemics.[16]

The inquiry to be headed by Lars Hedengran, head of law at the social affairs ministry since 2007, would take as its starting point the measures that had been implemented during the COVID-19 pandemic and the needs for these. During the pandemic, Hedengran had been involved in all legislative work related to pandemic management and this experience would be important in the work to develop a new infection control law adapted to future pandemics.[17]

The inquiry would review how to limit crowds to reduce the risk of spread and would analyse the need to link supervision and sanctions to the obligation of the individual to prevent the spread of infection. It would also review provisions for testing and tracing with the aim of formulating, in advance, practices that were better designed for a situation where needs greatly exceeded the normal.[18]

Tasks would include a review of extraordinary infection control measures such as looking at the possibility of taking samples from travellers entering Sweden or the possibility of temporary regional travel bans within Sweden. Careful consideration would have to be given to fundamental freedoms and rights of course, and any control measures should not go beyond what was necessary to prevent or counteract the spread of infection.[19]

Other tasks would include a review of how infection control could be strengthened for those in the care of social services, particularly those groups requiring special housing.[20]

The work of the inquiry on extraordinary control measures would have to reach conclusions in a partial report – a first inquiry report – on 15 May 2022, and the commission report finalised no later than 31 August 2023.[21]

Reopening of Sweden – Lifting of Restrictions – Trouble With Spikevax (Moderna)

At end-September 2021, nearly all of Sweden's pandemic restrictions and recommendations had been lifted, with 29 September marked by some as the 'day of freedom'.

There would no longer be any legal limits on distancing between tables in restaurants and bars, nor on sizes of groups sitting at them, though some establishments might continue to set their own rules. All restrictions on public events – limits on the number of attendees – had been removed too, paving the way for large concerts and sports matches, though again individual event organisers might set their own rules. Also lifted was the recommendation to work from home, though the public health agency advised employers to implement a phased or gradual return to the physical workplace. But of course, if an employee had symptoms they should always work from home and get tested, and the employer should take measures to assist working from home.[22]

After September however, those not vaccinated against COVID-19 were advised to keep a distance from people outside their closest circles, and to avoid close contact with people at risk and aged over 70. Because of the removal of rules ensuring distance at entertainment venues, they should avoid bars, nightclubs, theatres, concerts and sports events, where it would be difficult to keep distance.[23]

Even as the restrictions and recommendations were being lifted, from the public health agency Anders Tegnell reported that there had been a slight increase in deaths from the virus in recent weeks, though the number of new hospital admissions had fallen.[24]

While everyone had been longing for some kind of normality, and while for the world of sport, cultural life, and the hospitality industry, the lifting of restrictions had been vital, if not celebratory, the suffering could not be forgotten. Sweden had endured some 1.1 million confirmed cases of COVID-19, some 7,800 intensive care cases of the disease, and 14,800 deaths.[25]

The ongoing vaccination programme played an important part in the drive towards normality and the lifting of restrictions, but in early-October the public health agency had halted the use of the Moderna vaccine for the under-30s –

people born in 1991 and after. Analysis from Swedish and Nordic data had indicated a connection between Spikevax (the name given to the Moderna vaccine) and an increased incidence of heart inflammation, mainly in adolescents and young adults, and principally in boys and men. Only Comirnaty (the name given to the Pfizer/BioNTech vaccine) would now be administered to this age group.[26]

In Region Gävleborg, health authorities stopped the use of Spikevax for all age groups, saying they had enough Comirnaty to meet needs.[27]

Differing Guidance for Vaccinated and Unvaccinated – Booster Shots Begin

During October, the public health agency announced a change to COVID-19 guidance which would take effect from 1 November.

Although coronavirus infection continued to spread in Sweden, it was now at a stable level and relatively low compared with earlier months, and the country had achieved good vaccination coverage with some 80 per cent of the over-40s having received two doses. As a result, those who were fully vaccinated would no longer need to be tested if they had COVID-19 symptoms. They could return to work or study when they felt fit and had been fever-free for 24-hours, even if other symptoms persisted. For the unvaccinated, it would still be necessary to test for coronavirus, and testing and tracing would continue to apply to those working in elderly care and in healthcare. Travellers who had been to a country outside the Nordic region, regardless of whether or not they had been vaccinated, would also continue to be tested.[28]

The board of health and welfare (*Socialstyrelsen*) had also pointed out that seasonal flu, the winter vomiting bug, and other infections, were just around the corner and that it would be extra important to carry on with hygiene routines and other infection control measures. Additionally, just like before the pandemic, the advice was to stay at home in the event of illness or fever and only return to normal activity when fit and well. And, for everyone working in healthcare and in the care of the elderly, it was important that they carried out that care in a safe manner.[29]

Also in October, Hallengren and Johan Carlson announced that everyone over the age of sixty-five would be offered a third COVID-19 vaccine dose, a booster. Nursing home residents, those getting care at home, and all over-80s, had already been eligible for a booster. Eventually everyone over 16 would be offered one, and for that wider population it would be rolled out over the winter and spring. It would be up to the regions to decide how to administer the vaccination programmes.[30]

Statistics, October–November 2021 – Among Lowest Infection Spread in Europe – 5,000,000 COVID-19 Deaths Around the World

Well into October, the spread of COVID-19 infection in Sweden had been recorded at 55.36 daily new confirmed cases per million in a 7-day rolling average, which at the time was among the lowest in Europe (20 October 2021). At the height of summer, very much lower spread had been recorded on some days too – 20.8 cases on that measure on 13 July.[31]

The spread on that day in October had been significantly lower than in almost all other European countries and certainly those in Sweden's near neighbourhood of Baltic and Nordic Europe. Latvia had 1,180.78 daily new confirmed COVID-19 cases per million people on that day, Lithuania 971.27, Estonia 857.45, Iceland 167.73, Germany 146.66, Denmark 133.83, Finland 88.24, and Norway 81.86. In the UK it was 664.47, in the USA 231.32, and in Brazil 55.9.[32]

Only San Marino, Italy, Spain, Malta, Kosovo, and Vatican City had a lower spread of infection on that day, with San Marino recording 46.2 daily new confirmed cases per million on a 7-day rolling average, Italy 44.49, Spain 40, Malta 31.28, Kosovo 8.66, and Vatican City none.[33]

High vaccination coverage in Sweden and the advanced healthcare system had accounted for the low spread of infection. However, what could not be accounted for now, was why in Norway say, there had been major outbreaks in schools affecting both students and teachers, unlike in the earlier stages of the pandemic. Although it had not yet happened in Sweden, it suggested that the virus was moving in a different way, which was surprising since schools had not been a risky environment before.

Tegnell said that the key to keeping the spread of infection down would be to continue vaccinating people in their 20s to 40s because they were the age group likely to drive the spread of infection. He added that with such a low spread of infection, there was a risk that willingness would weaken, and that fewer people would choose to get their first or second injection. The country had to continue to get vaccinated otherwise there was a high probability that spread would take off again. If there were a new wave throughout the country, it could bring about renewed restrictions across Sweden. Another concern was the autumn holiday and unnecessary travel to countries from which there was a high risk of importing infection.

As far as the spread of infection was concerned, Sweden was at a pronounced plateau statistically at end-October, with newly confirmed cases neither going up nor down. The curve was very flat and had been since the relaxation of restrictions.

By 1 November 2021, the global death toll from COVID-19 had passed 5,000,000. Of these, 1.3 million had occurred in Europe, 1.18 million in Asia, 1.17 million in South America, 1.13 million in North America, 218,234 in Africa, and 1,743 in Australia. In Sweden 15,025 had died, in Denmark 2,714, in Finland 1,158, in Norway 900, and in Iceland 33.[34]

Of the deaths in Europe, Russia had accounted for 234,194, the UK 141,735, and Italy 132,100. Relative to population, Bosnia and Herzegovina had recorded the greatest number of deaths per million people with 3,522.34, while Bulgaria had recorded 3,479.8, and Montenegro 3,189.59. The statistics for the EU were 796,951 cumulative deaths and 1,782.13 per million.[35]

Of the deaths in Asia, India had accounted for 458,437, Indonesia 143,405, and Iran 126,303. Relative to population, Armenia had recorded the greatest number of deaths per million with 2,131.98, while Iran had recorded 1,485.41, and Lebanon 1,255.99.[36]

Of the deaths in South America, Brazil had accounted for 608,082, Peru 200,246, and Colombia 127,281. Relative to population, Peru had recorded the greatest number of deaths per million people with 6,002.68, while Brazil had recorded 2,841.59, and Argentina 2,542.44.[37]

Of the deaths in North America, and including Central America, the USA had accounted for 747,358, Mexico 288,365, and Canada 29,022. Relative to population, the USA had recorded the greatest number of deaths per million people with 2,244.89, while Mexico had recorded 2,213.73, and Grenada 1,751.98.[38]

Of the deaths in Africa, South Africa had accounted for 89,177, Tunisia 25,241, and Egypt 18,651. Relative to population, Tunisia had recorded the greatest number of deaths per million people with 2,114.74, while South Africa had recorded 1,485,24, and Namibia 1,373.61.[39]

Of the deaths in Australia, New Zealand, Oceania and Fiji, Oceania had accounted for 3,724, Australia 1,743, Fiji 674, and New Zealand 28. Relative to population, Fiji had recorded the greatest number of deaths per million people with 746.48, while Oceania had recorded 86.16, Australia 67.59, and New Zealand 5.47.[40]

Taken together, the toll in the EU (796,951) the USA (747,358), Brazil (608,082), and the UK (140,735), had accounted for almost half the worldwide deaths (2,293,126), and yet the same countries only accounted for one eighth of the world's population. One explanation for this was the composition of these populations. Wealthier countries often had a higher life expectancy and therefore a larger proportion of older citizens – the group that was at high risk of suffering from serious illness. In poorer countries, it was children and young people that made up the larger proportion of citizens.[41]

Despite wealthier countries having advanced healthcare systems, these were not always enough. COVID-19 was a disease that affected the very oldest the hardest and so it was hardly surprising that countries with a larger proportion of older people had recorded high mortality and stretched healthcare services and intensive care units. Regardless of what healthcare did, it was not possible to save all lives. Even advanced healthcare systems become heavily burdened when a lot of people fall ill at the same time.[42]

Then there was the link between death rates and prosperity within individual countries. Less well-off areas often accounted for large parts of both the spread of infection and death. Risk factors for COVID-19 were more common among vulnerable groups – a pattern seen for many other diseases – and could be about factors such as smoking, obesity, or untreated diabetes.[43]

Vaccine Passes For Public Gatherings and Events

In November, Karin Tegmark Wisell took over as the new director-general of the public health agency replacing Johan Carlson who had retired at the end of October.

At a press conference, Tegmark Wisell explained that from 1 December 2021 vaccine passes would be required to access all indoor public gatherings and public events of more than 100 attendees – at theatres, concerts, cinemas, nightclubs, sports events, dance performances, funfairs and amusement parks, demonstrations, and religious services. Outdoor events such as Christmas markets and funfairs would not require a vaccine pass, nor would indoor events of less than 100 attendees. Restaurants and bars were not being subjected to the vaccine pass requirement either unless they organized some kind of music or dance entertainment drawing over 100 people. If infections rose dramatically this could change. Classes and lectures at school or university were not classified as public gatherings or events either, nor were shops, workplaces, and public transport services.[44]

From politicians in Stockholm and Region Skåne had come calls for the use of vaccine passes across wider society, and for those who had been double vaccinated. Expansion of their use would encourage more people to get vaccinated and ensure that society remained open. Those who had acted responsibly and been vaccinated ought to be able to move freely, especially as there was a risk of increased infection over the coming winter months.[45]

New Omicron-Variant

Towards end-November came concerning news from South Africa of a heavily mutated version of COVID-19. The confirmed cases were still mostly concentrated in one province, but there were hints that it could have spread further.[46]

South Africa had first reported the COVID-19 variant (B.1.1.529) to the WHO on 24 November. The recent epidemiological situation in the country had been characterised by steeply increasing infections coinciding with the detection of the new variant. The first known confirmed infection was from a specimen collected on 9 November 2021.[47]

The evolution of SARS-CoV-2 was periodically monitored and evaluated by the Technical Advisory Group on SARS-CoV-2 Virus Evolution (TAG-VE), and the body was also tasked with assessing whether specific mutations and combinations of mutations altered the behaviour of the virus. On 26 November, TAG-VE was convened to assess the SARS-CoV-2 variant. Subsequently, and based on evidence that was 'indicative of a detrimental change in COVID-19 epidemiology', the TAG-VE had advised the WHO that B.1.1.529 should be designated as a 'variant of concern', and on 26 November, the WHO duly named it the Omicron-variant.[48]

The response to the Omicron-variant was immediate, and stock markets were affected, though they did stabilize. A few days later however, Stéphane Bancel, the CEO of Moderna Pharmaceuticals, had cast doubts on the effectiveness of vaccines against the new variant, and markets around the world again fell. He predicted that existing vaccines would be less effective in staving off the Omicron-variant, and that it would take months for pharmaceutical companies to update vaccines.[49]

News about the variant prompted a meeting of EU health experts, and following on from that, EU member states decided to impose temporary restrictions on air travel from southern Africa. Von der Leyen said that the decision had been taken until more was known about the variant. The UK stopped all direct flights from six countries in southern Africa: South Africa, Lesotho, Botswana, Zimbabwe, Mozambique, Namibia, and Eswatini. The Netherlands, Czechia, and Italy also announced that they were stopping flights from South Africa. Denmark stopped unnecessary travel to South Africa and several other African countries. Germany announced that only German citizens were allowed to enter from the countries, and they had to be quarantined. Israel, Canada, India, the United States and a number of other countries also introduced various measures. Sweden had no direct flights from South Africa.[50]

Tegnell said that Sweden already recommended that those coming from southern Africa should get tested, and now the recommendation would be extended to any arrivals who were already vaccinated. Travellers arriving in Sweden from southern Africa were encouraged to stay at home for a week, regardless of whether they had symptoms or not. Tegnell urged anyone planning on going to South Africa to think about their decision. Disregarding the risk imposed by the Omicron-variant itself, travel to the country would be difficult, as would the return journey. It was a bad time to be travelling.[51]

A good deal more upbeat than Moderna's Bancel, Sweden's vaccine coordinator, Richard Bergström, had said that if vaccines did require adjustment to protect against the Omicron-variant, pharmaceutical companies could do this within three months of a decision by authorities. Additionally, Europe's entire requirement for mRNA vaccines was now satisfied from its own production. Europe was self-sufficient, all its manufacture happened there, and Sweden was able to access the supply. During the first half of 2022, Sweden had contracts for 9.5 million doses of the Pfizer/BioNTech vaccine and a further 11 million for the next six months. In addition, Moderna would deliver 9 million doses during the year. If required to be, all the doses would be modified to protect against the new Omicron-variant.[52]

Statistics, December 2021

As the second year of the COVID-19 pandemic drew to a close, cumulative deaths across the Nordic countries had been recorded on 31 December 2021 as: in Sweden 15,310, Denmark 3,267, Finland 1,564, Norway 1,305, and in Iceland 37.[53]

While Sweden's figures clearly had been very much worse than those of close neighbours, they stood up well in comparison to those recorded in Portugal, Czechia, Greece, and Hungary. Not greatly different from Sweden in terms of population size (Portugal, Czechia, and Greece were slightly larger), cumulatively Portugal had recorded 18,955 deaths, while Greece and Czechia had recorded 20,790 and 36,129 deaths respectively. Hungary, slightly smaller than Sweden population-wise had recorded 39,186 deaths. Czechia and Hungary had recorded more than twice as many deaths as Sweden. Relative to population at end-December, Sweden's recorded deaths had been 1,506.87 per million, whereas Portugal had recorded 1,864.2, Greece 2,004.68, Czechia 3,368.81, and Hungary 4,067.4. Cumulatively since the start of the pandemic, the UK had recorded 2,180.67 deaths per million, and the USA 2,480.45.[54] Was Sweden still the outlier?

Russia, the UK, Italy, France, Germany, and Ukraine had recorded the highest number of cumulative deaths by end-December, each country recording between 100,000 and 300,000 victims. In Russia the figure was 302,671 and in the UK 148,737, the milestone of 140,000 UK deaths having been passed 26–27 October. In Italy the number of deaths had been 137,402, in France 123,805, in Germany 112,111, and in Ukraine 102,088. In China, where the virus had been first identified, there had been only 4,636 deaths claimed since January 2020, though only 2 additional deaths since 12 January 2021 beggared belief.[55]

Cumulatively worldwide, some 5.44 million people had died from COVID-19 since January 2020. In the continent of Europe, there had been 1.53 million deaths since then, and in the EU, 904,340. In Asia there had been 1.26 million deaths, in North America 1.22 million, in South America 1.19 million, in Africa 227,907, and in Australia 2,248.[56]

As far as vaccinations were concerned, by end-December 2021, the share of the Swedish population fully vaccinated against COVID-19, with all doses prescribed by the vaccination protocol was 72.85 per cent. Those having at least one dose of COVID-19 vaccine was 76.25 per cent. By way of comparison, in the UK 69.54 per cent were fully vaccinated, in Norway 71.75 per cent, Finland 74.75 per cent, Iceland 76.99, and Denmark 78.69 per cent. In the UK 75.93 per cent had at least one dose of vaccine, in Iceland 78.16 per cent, in Norway 78.4 per cent, Finland 78.41 per cent, and in Denmark 82.65 per cent.[57]

The total number of vaccine booster doses administered per 100 people across the Nordic countries end-December 2021 were: in Iceland 54.48 boosters, in Denmark 48.29, in Norway 28.51, in Sweden 25.29, Finland 20.41.[58]

In the UK it had been 49.98, in Israel 45.74, in the USA 21.71, in Brazil 12.42, and in Russia 5.06.[59]

Towards the Year End, 2021

In a statement by Hans Kluge, WHO regional director, on 21 December, the Omicron-variant had been detected in thirty-eight of the fifty-three member states of the WHO European Region since its first detection less than a month earlier.[60]

The variant had become dominant in several countries, including Denmark, Portugal, and the UK, and had been transmitted mostly among adults in their 20s and 30s, and had spread initially in large cities and in social and workplace gatherings. Countries had to protect, prevent, and prepare.[61]

Ahead of Christmas, as the spread of the Omicron-variant became concerning, and with the prospect of pressure on the healthcare system, the Swedish government and public health agency announced new measures. Everyone who could do so was to work from home, and in restaurants there would be a return to table service only with one metre distance between groups. Shopping centres, and cultural and leisure facilities, would have to re-introduce measures to limit crowding. Until more people had received their booster vaccinations, plans to extend the vaccine pass system for entry to restaurants and long-distance public transport had been put on hold. Public events for more than twenty people would have to have assigned seating, and public events of more than 500 would have to request vaccine passes for admission, hold groups to a maximum of eight, and maintain distancing between groups. There was to be no partying in night clubs on New Year's Eve.[62]

On 29 December, at a press conference, Ghebreyesus, director-general of the WHO, said that the older Delta-variant and the new Omicron-variant had become a twin threat to the world. The variants were driving up cases to record numbers and again leading to spikes in hospitalisation and deaths. The ideal conditions for their emergence had been created by populism, and narrow nationalism, and the undermining of equity by a small number of countries that had hoarded health tools such as masks, therapeutics, diagnostics, and vaccines. He said that science and trust in lifesaving health tools had been distracted and undermined by misinformation and disinformation, often spread by a small number of people. This had driven vaccine hesitancy, translating into the unvaccinated dying disproportionally. The virus, he said, would continue to evolve and threaten health systems unless there was an improvement in the collective response. He voiced his concern that Omicron being more transmissible, circulating at the same time as Delta, was 'leading to a tsunami of cases'.[63]

Chapter 10 focusses on the committee of inquiry into the spread of COVID-19, the *Coronakommission*, and its first interim report, as well as the work of the parliamentary standing committee on the constitution (*Konstitutionsutskottet, KU*) which had been questioning ministers, agency directors, and others, on the actions they had taken to deal with the pandemic. Could the opposition have done any better in handling the crisis? Additionally, the COVID-related Budget Bill, and new pandemic law are looked at. How much had the country's mitigation measures cost?

Notes

1 'In numbers: Covid-19 cases continue to rise in Sweden', *The Local*, 12 August 2021, <https://www.thelocal.se/20210812/in-numbers-covid-19-cases-continue-to-rise-in-sweden/> accessed 21 August 2021.

2 Lallerstedt, Siri. 'Det här är pandemilagen och tillfälliga serveringslag', *Dagens Nyheter*, 12 August 2021, <https://www.dn.se/sverige/det-har-ar-pandemilagen-och-tillfalliga-serveringslagen/> accessed 21 August 2021.

3 'National Union of Teachers calls on Sweden to vaccinate children against Covid', The Local, 16 August 2021, <https://www.thelocal.se/20210816/national-union-of-teachers-calls-on-sweden-to-vaccinate-children-against-covid/> accessed 31 August 2021.

4 Bjurwald, Lisa. 'Opinion: I believe Sweden will regret its approach to COVID in schools', *The Local*, 16 August 2021, <https://www.thelocal.se/20210816/opinion-i-believe-sweden-will-regret-its-approach-to-covid-in-schools/> accessed 31 August 2021.

5 'Efter tantrafestivalen – Norge rödmarkerar Värmland igen', *SVT Nyheter*, Värmland, 13 August 2021, updated 17 August 2021, <https://www.svt.se/nyheter/lokalt/varmland/norks-regeringen-meddelar-varmland-blir-ater-rott> accessed 21 August 2021.

6 Löfgren, Emma. 'Sweden in violation of EU law for failing to issue COVID passes to thousands of foreign residents', *The Local*, 25 August 2021, updated 29 August 2021, <https://www.thelocal.se/20210825/sweden-in-violation-of-eu-law-for-failing-to-issue-covid-passes-to-everyone/> accessed 31 August 2021.

7 'E-hälsomyndigheten ska undersöka om fler vaccinerade grupper kan få covidbevis', Press release, Ministry of Social Affairs, Regeringskansliet/Government Offices of Sweden, 26 August 2021, <https://www.regeringen.se/pressmeddelanden/2021/08/e-halsomyndigheten-ska-undersoka-om-fler-vaccinerade-grupper-kan-fa-covidbevis/> accessed 29 September 2021.

The eHealth Agency advised those vaccinated in another EU country to obtain that country's version of the COVID pass, and recommended that the government appoint one national authority to be responsible for authorizing foreign (non-EU) vaccinations.

8 'Sweden to roll out Covid pass to remaining groups by year end', *The Local*, 28 October 2021, <https://www.thelocal.se/20211028/Sweden-to-roll-out-covid-pass-to-remaining-groups-by-year-end/> accessed 6 November 2021.

9 'Vaccinated travellers to Sweden from the UK to be exempted from entry ban and test requirement', Ministry of Justice, Government Offices of Sweden, 7 October 2021, <https://www.government.se/press-releases/2021/10/vaccinated-travellers-to-sweden-from-the-uk-to-be-exempted-from-entry-ban-and-test-requirement/> accessed 10 October 2021.

10 'Øresundsbron bjuder på turer för att omstarta regionen', Øresundsbron website, 31 August 2021, <https://www.oresundsbron.com/sv/info/omstart> accessed 29 September 2021. The Øresund Bridge had been a joint project undertaken by Denmark and Sweden, and the completed bridge was owned and operated by Øresundsbro Konsortiet, jointly owned by the Danish and Swedish states. The formal name of the bridge is Øresundsbron, a Scandinavian 'hybrid word' merging the Danish rendering of Øresundsbroen with the Swedish Öresundsbron.

11 Ibid.

12 Ibid.

13 'How Denmark plans to attract more workers from Sweden', *The Local*, 20 October 2021, <https://www.thelocal.se/20211020/how-denmark-plans-to-attract-more-workers-from-sweden/> accessed 24 October 2021.

14 Norwell, Frazer. 'Oslo to Gothenburg train service set to make a return', *The Local*, 3 September 2021, <https://www.thelocal.se/20210903/oslo-to-gothenburg-train-service-set-to-return-to-the-rails/> accessed 3 October 2021.

15 'Stockholm-Oslo train service set to resume', *The Local*, 7 October 2021, <https://www.thelocal.se/20211007/stockholm-oslo-train-service-set-to-resume/> accessed 9 October 2021.

16 'Utredning ska se över smittskyddslagen inför framtida pandemier, Press release, Socialdepartementet / Ministry of Social Affairs, Regeringskansliet / Government Offices of Sweden, 31 August 2021, <https://www.regeringen.se/pressmeddelanden/2021/08/utredning-ska-se-over-smittskyddslagen-infor-framtida-pandemier/> accessed 2 October 2021.

17 Ibid.

18 Ibid.

19 Ibid.

20 Ibid.

21 Ibid.

22 'Key points: How Sweden's Covid-19 rules change today', *The Local*, 8 September, updated 29 September 2021, <https://www.thelocal.se/20210908/key-points-how-swedens-covid-19-restrictions-will-change-at-the-end-of-the-month/> accessed 4 October 2021.

23 Ibid.

24 'Coronavirus: The latest news about the outbreak in Sweden', *The Local*, 2 September 2020, updated 30 September, <https://www.thelocal.se/20200902/coronavirus-the-latest-news-about-the-outbreak-in-sweden-timeline-part-two/> accessed 4 October 2021.

25 Lundberg, Patrik. 'Nu firar vi medelklassens frihetsdag', *Dagens Nyheter*, 28 September 2021, <https://www.dn.se/sverige/patrik-lundberg-nu-firar-vi-medelklassens-frihetsdag/> accessed 4 October 2021.

26 Bratt, Anna. 'Därför stoppas bara Modernas vaccin', *Dagens Nyheter*, 6 October 2021, updated 7 October 2021, <https://www.dn.se/vetenskap/anna-bratt-darfor-stoppas-bara-modernas-vaccin/> accessed 10 October 2021.

[27] Olsson, Gustav. 'Gävleborg pausar Moderna helt—behöver inte längre vaccinet', *Dagens Nyheter*, 7 October 2021, <https://www.dn.se/sverige/gavleborg-pausar-moderna-helt-behover-inte-langre-vaccinet/> accessed 10 October 2021.

[28] Linder, Julia. and Sofia Tanaka, and Mia Holmgren. 'FHM:s nya riktlinjer efter första november: Vaccinerade behöver inte testa sig', *Dagens Nyheter*, 14 October 2021, <https://www.dn.se/sverige.fhms-nya-riktlinjer-efter-forsta-november-vaccinerade-behover-inte-testa-sig/> accessed 15 October 2021.

[29] Ibid.

[30] 'Sweden rolls out Covid-19 booster shot to over-65s', *The Local*, 27 October 2021, <https://www.thelocal.se/20211027/sweden-rolls-out-covid-19-booster-shot-to-over-65s/> accessed 6 November 2021.

[31] 'Daily new confirmed COVID-19 cases per million people, October 20, 2021', Our World in Data, COVID-19 dataset, <https://ourworldindata.org> accessed 15 January 2022.

[32] Ibid.

[33] Ibid.

[34] 'Cumulative confirmed COVID-19 deaths, Oct 31, 2021, Our World in Data, COVID- 19 dataset, <https://ourworldindata.org> accessed 15 January 2022.

[35] 'Cumulative confirmed COVID-19 deaths, Oct 31, 2021' & 'Cumulative confirmed COVID-19deaths per million, Oct 31, 2021, Our World in Data, COVID-19 dataset, <https://ourworldindata.org> accessed 15 January 2022.

[36] Ibid.

[37] Ibid.

[38] Ibid.

[39] Ibid.

[40] Ibid.

[41] Olsson, Gustav. 'Världen passerar fem miljoner dödsfall – rika länder hårt drabbade', *Dagens Nyheter*, 1 November 2021, <https://www.dn.se/varlden/varlden-passerar-fem-miljoner-dodsfall-rika-lander-hart-drabbade/> accessed 2 November 2021.

[42] Ibid.

[43] Ibid.

[44] Waterton, Becky. 'Which events will require Sweden's new vaccine pass?', *The Local*, 18 November 2021, <https://www.thelocal.se/20211118/which-events-will-require-swedens-new-vaccine-pass/> accessed 18 November 2021.

[45] Waterton, Becky. 'Swedish politicians call for Covid vaccine pass requirement', *The Local*, 16 November 2021, <https://www.thelocal.se/20211116/swedish-politicians-call-for-covid-vaccine-pass-requirement/> accessed 18 November 2021.

[46] Gallagher, James. 'New COVID variant: How worried should we be?' *BBC News*, 26 November 2021, <https://www.bbc.co.uk/news/health-59418127> accessed 30 November 2021.

[47] 'Classification of Omicron (B.1.1.529): SARS-CoV-2 Variant of Concern', News, World Health Organization (WHO), 26 November 2021, <https://www.who.int/news/item/26-11-2021-classification-of-omicron-(b.1.1.529)-sars-cov-2-variant-of-concern> accessed 30 November 2021.

[48] Ibid.

[49] 'Global markets fall after Moderna Omicron warning', *BBC News*, 30 November 2021, <https://www.bbc.co.uk/news/business-59426353> accessed 30 November 2021.

[50] Svahn, Clas. 'Sverige kan ha modifierat vaccin inom tre månader', *Dagens Nyheter*, 26 November 2021, updated 27 November 2021, <https://www.dn.se/sverige/sverige-kan-ha-modifierat-vaccin-inom-tre-manader/> accessed 30 November 2021.

[51] Ibid.

52 Ibid.

53 'Cumulative confirmed COVID-19 deaths, December 31, 2021', Our World in Data, COVID-19 dataset, <https://ourworldindata.org> accessed 16 January 2022.

54 Ibid., and 'Cumulative confirmed COVID-19 deaths per million people, December 31, 2021', Our World in Data, COVID-19 dataset, <https://ourworldindata.org> accessed 16 January 2022.

55 'Cumulative confirmed COVID-19 deaths, December 31, 2021', as note 53.

56 Ibid.

57 'COVID-19 vaccine doses, people with at least one dose, people fully vaccinated, and boosters per 100 people, December 31, 2021', Our World in Data, COVID-19 dataset, <https://ourworldindata.org> accessed 16 January 2022.

58 Ibid.

59 Ibid.

60 'Statement – Update on Covid-19: Omicron is gaining ground: Protect, prevent, prepare', Statement by Dr. Hans Henri P. Kluge, WHO Regional Director for Europe, WHO, Regional Office for Europe, 21 December 2021, <https://www.euro.who.int/en/media-centre/sections/statements/2021/statement-update-on-covid-19-omicron-is-gaining-ground-protect,-prevent,-prepare> accessed 22 December 2021.

61 Ibid.

62 'We must adapt to the new reality: Sweden rolls out new COVID measures', *The Local*, 21 December 2021, <https://www.thelocal.se/20211221/we-must-adapt-to-the-new-reality-sweden-rolls-out-new-covid-measures/> accessed 22 December 2021.

63 'WHO director-general's opening remarks at the press conference – 29 December 2021', WHO, 29 December 2021, <https://www.who.int/director-general/speeches/detail/who-director-general-s-opening-remarks-at-the-press-conference---29-december-2021> accessed 30 December 2021.

Coronakommissionen and Other Inquiries

Committee of Inquiry into the Spread of COVID-19 – *Coronakommissionen*

In the face of growing criticism from the opposition during the summer and of falling public confidence in the ability of the government to handle COVID-19 – not least as regards the care of the elderly – the government announced that a committee of inquiry into the spread of coronavirus across the health and social care sector was to be set up.

Answering the criticism, Lena Hallengren, the health and social affairs minister, had said that the government had been prepared at all times to introduce further and wider measures recommended by experts. For his part, prime minister Stefan Löfven had admitted that although the overall strategy of limiting the disease while also protecting workers and companies had been correct, when it came to care of the elderly and the spread of infection, Sweden had fallen down somewhat.[1]

In May 2020, and under continuing pressure from the opposition, the prime minister let it be known that a committee of inquiry would be set up to investigate the spread of COVID-19.[2]

The Moderates and the Sweden Democrats had called for a commission to be in place before the summer, and though Löfven expressed his support for one, he had said initially that it would be appointed after the pandemic was over. On 30 June however, a committee had been appointed with the formal remit of evaluating the measures taken by the government, administrative authorities, and municipalities, to limit the spread of the virus that caused COVID-19, and the effects of its spread. It was to examine how the crisis management organisation at government level, in administrative agencies, and in regions and municipalities had worked during the pandemic. The commission would also evaluate how the principle of responsibility and geographical responsibility for specific areas had worked during the crisis, and it was to propose measures based on its observations.[3]

The inquiry would also conduct an international comparison with other relevant countries of the various measures that Sweden had taken since the start of the pandemic.[4]

The remit would not be too far removed from that of the inquiry set up in the UK later to examine the response to, and the impact of, the COVID-19 pandemic in the UK, and to produce a factual narrative account. The UK COVID-19 Inquiry began its public hearings in June 2023 and would identify lessons to be learned and inform the preparations for future pandemics. Anders Tegnell would submit a witness testimony to the British inquiry.

The Swedish commission was to be chaired by Mats Melin, appointed by the government. A justice and president of the Supreme Administrative Court (*Högsta förvaltningsdomstolen*) between 2011 and 2018, and chief parliamentary ombudsman (*Riksdagens ombudsman*) 2004 and 2011, Melin had participated in several central government inquiries before, including the committee 1991–93 that investigated constitutional amendments needed prior to joining the EU. He had also served at the Court of Justice of the EU.[5]

The inquiry was to submit its final report by the end of February 2022, but before then it would present two interim reports (*delbetänkande*), one in November 2020 with a focus on 'Elderly care during the pandemic', and the second in October 2021 with a focus on 'Sweden during the pandemic'.[6]

The final report would be published a full seven months before the 2022 General Election.

In the meantime, a report by the Health and Social Care Inspectorate (*Inspektionen för vård och omsorg, IVO*) which came out in November had been highly critical of the treatment of some care home residents during the pandemic and had highlighted how some patients had died without ever having been given an assessment by a doctor. Serious flaws in the care of the elderly could not only be blamed on coronavirus but had existed even without taking the pandemic into account. The minimum level of care had been simply too low, even during a pandemic.[7]

First Interim Report – *Coronakommissionen*

The first of the interim reports of Melin's Corona Commission came out on 7 December, rather than in November. Its focus had been 'Elderly care during the pandemic'.

In brief, it found that Sweden had failed to protect care home residents from the coronavirus, and that the government was to blame for this. Other individual agencies and authorities bore responsibility as well. Notwithstanding the general spread of the virus across Sweden, the factor having the greatest impact on the number of cases and deaths from the virus in the residential care sector were the structural shortcomings that had been well known for a long time. These had led to the sector being unprepared and ill-equipped to handle a pandemic. Staff employed in elderly and residential care had been largely left by themselves to tackle the crisis.[8]

The report had also noted that Sweden had not suffered an especially high share of deaths in care homes as a proportion of total COVID-19 fatalities, when compared to other countries. However, the protection of the elderly – an age group known to be particularly vulnerable to serious illness from COVID-19 – had been a key tenet of the Swedish pandemic response.[9]

It found that the main factor among the problems faced by residential elderly care homes had been the fact that the virus had spread so widely in society. But other factors were highlighted. Measures put in place in the spring had come just too late and, although it was known that the elderly and care home residents were a vulnerable group, they were insufficient. For example, the ban on visiting care homes ought to have been in place earlier than it had been, and there should have been an explicit exception made for end-of-life visits. The fact that many people had died without a relative by their side was unacceptable, even if the ban had been motivated as part of the strategy for limiting the spread of the virus.[10]

There had been other findings. The report pointed out structural issues that had been raised by both the OECD and the WHO even before the pandemic, namely, low levels of staffing and expertise. The commission proposed that this be reviewed and particularly called for fewer zero-hours contracts. PPE (or personal protective equipment) was also raised as an issue – the fact that there had been limited amounts of PPE. The report showed that two government agencies had noted in early-February that there was a risk of a possible lack of protective equipment, however the board of health and welfare had only begun preparing an overview of the situation in the various municipalities in April. This had been long after the virus had entered the residential and elderly care sector. The report also criticised the public health agency for only publishing its national testing strategy seventeen days after it had been urged to do so by the government.[11]

Finally, it had been the assessment of the inquiry that central government agencies did not have enough of an overview of the problems and deficiencies in municipal elderly care, and even if specific agencies had been directly responsible for different elements of the strategy, the government held overall responsibility.

The ultimate responsibility rested with the government in power – Löfven and the centre-left coalition – but also with those previous governments that had possessed knowledge of the structural shortcomings in elderly care.[12]

Löfven's Response

Following the presentation of the first interim report of the Corona Commission, Löfven said that he agreed with its findings.

The 'harsh criticism' from the commission had, as he saw it, 'been reasonable'. The infection had spread quickly through the care homes with many cases and deaths, and when restrictions were introduced on visiting, this affected both the elderly and their relatives. It had been 'a miserable time'. The commission had been correct in its criticism of elderly care. Sweden's pandemic tragedy had been played out in its care homes 'where so many old people died, sometimes under difficult circumstances, alone, separated from relatives and friends'.[13]

His response to the first interim report was to launch a media offensive placing the shortcomings on his political opponents in local government.[14]

Löfven's media offensive focussed on how the responsibility for failures in the protection of the elderly had been apportioned across his own government, previous governments, municipal government, and regional government, but rather than taking the blame himself or laying it on his own ministers, or the public health agency or Tegnell, he homed in on the commission's criticism of municipal and regional government.[15]

He pushed the narrative that the eight Alliance years between 2006 and 2014 had seen reduction in the funding for elderly care leaving it vulnerable to the pandemic. He zeroed in on the role of locally elected officials who steered much of the health and elderly care system, many of whom represented opposition parties, including those currently running Stockholm. This narrative allowed him to say that Sweden needed to rebuild its welfare system, the area in which the electorate trusted the Social Democrats most.[16] Nevertheless, critics could justifiably argue that the party had had six years since 2014 to fix things.

KU and Its Investigation of Sweden's Handling of the Pandemic

The second interim report – expected in autumn 2021 – would be eagerly anticipated of course, but in addition to Melin's inquiry, and that of the Health and Social Care Inspectorate reporting the previous November, the parliamentary Standing Committee on the Constitution (*Konstitutionsutskottet, KU*) had also been questioning ministers, agency directors, and others, on the actions they had taken to deal with the pandemic. Regarded as the most powerful of Sweden's permanent standing committees, one of its tasks was to examine the performance of the prime minister and how the government handled important issues.[17]

The committee had been led by Karin Enström, from the Moderates, a former defence minister (2012–14). Its remit was to go beyond the narrow area being investigated by the Corona Commission (which was looking at elderly care) and to examine five broader areas: the decisions taken by the government on strategy; whether the government had properly grounded its decisions on factual evidence; whether government communication around strategy been correct and clear; whether government crisis management and crisis leadership had been in accordance with the precautionary principle; and whether the government should have had a better constitutional readiness. The committee had the power to call anybody for questioning, and in addition to grilling Carlson, the investigation had questioned Anders Knape, the chair of the Swedish Association of Local Authorities and Regions, SALAR (or *Sveriges Kommuner och Regioner*), Harriet Wallberg, the former national coronavirus testing coordinator, and Olivia Wigzell, general director of the board of health and welfare.[18]

In March 2021, Dan Eliasson, former head of the Civil Contingencies Agency (the MSB), sat before the committee. He stated that as early as February 2020 his agency had wanted to sound the alarm about the risks that Sweden faced from coronavirus. A report had been laid before the justice ministry on 6 February warning of serious shortages in personal protective equipment (PPE), and the MSB had frequently advocated for faster and more comprehensive measures including digital contact-tracing. There had been a number of situations where the MSB would have wanted to see more and earlier measures, said Eliasson. He acknowledged however that it was in the very nature of his agency to be a constant prophet of doom – offering scenarios that rarely if ever came to pass – and that it should always expect a negative response from ministries and other bodies.[19]

Carlson denied that the MSB had questioned the strategy of the public health agency and said that while there had been discussions over scrapping the planned contact-tracing app there had not been any broader criticisms. He claimed that essentially the Swedish strategy had not been any different from that of any other European country, adding that it had remained constant throughout the pandemic. What differed were the measures used by countries to push down the level of infection, and where Sweden had been correct was in the decision not to impose the drastic levels of lockdown imposed elsewhere.[20]

Government ministers, including Löfven, Hallengren, and Mikael Damberg the home affairs minister, were questioned by the *KU* investigation during April and May. Indeed, it was a humble prime minister that had appeared before the investigation. 'Sweden had been hard hit, and we should make no secret of that', Löfven had said in April.[21]

Löfven had defended his management of the crisis. When quizzed about herd immunity, he firmly rejected that goal as having been part of his strategy. 'Of course not', he said. 'Never, never ever'. The goal had always been to suppress the infection as far as possible. He did not however give any real explanation as to why his government had waited so long before putting in place several key measures against the spread of infection. Although COVID-19 had been classified as a disease constituting a danger to society on 1 February 2020, and an advisory on non-essential travel had been in place since 17 March, the recommendation on social distancing had not come until 1 April 2020. It had been autumn 2020 before stricter rules were introduced on public gatherings, and it was only recently that people had been expected to quarantine if somebody in the household was suspected of having become infected. Why had that not been in place last spring?[22] Hallengren and Damberg had also been questioned about the speed and timing of putting in place Sweden's measures.

The committee was expected to report in June 2021.

'Rare' Royal Opinion – Sweden's 'Failed' Approach

Coming after the publication of the first interim report of the Corona Commission, and viewed as a royal rebuke, Carl XIV Gustaf said that he believed the country had failed to save lives during the pandemic.[23] The comment had come in December in the wake of the report, and during an interview in a television review of the 'royal year' (for SVT), and from a monarch with largely ceremonial roles and who did not typically comment on political matters.

A large number of people had died, and that was terrible, the king had said. The people of Sweden had suffered tremendously in difficult conditions. He referred to all the family members who had been unable to say goodbye to their loved ones and to the grief and frustration in many families. 'I think it is a tough and traumatic experience not to be able to say a warm goodbye', he said. He also expressed his concern for those in business who were on their knees and could lose their livelihoods.[24]

A royal court spokesperson said that the king's remarks should not be taken as his comment on the strategy, and that they had been non-political. In referring to the country having 'failed', the king had been remarking on the whole of Sweden and the whole society, and not the government nor public agencies. He had been showing empathy and compassion towards those who had been affected in different ways, and to those who had died in the pandemic.[25]

Löfven said that he had interpreted the king's comments as 'confirmation' of what had already been said. The fact that so many people had died was a failure, and that could not be seen in any other way. That was how he interpreted it, he said. For his part, Tegnell did not want to comment on the king's criticism. What had been success or failure would be talked about for a long time to come. While he said it was obvious that the number of deaths in Sweden was deeply regrettable, he would not be drawn on the question of whether he thought the king was right, saying that it should be left to those researching and investigating the strategy in the future to take a stand on. He had no opinion on what the king said or thought.[26]

No stranger to controversy over the years, the king's comments had attracted a great deal of international attention. And why wouldn't it? After all, the king's comments on Sweden having 'failed' simply fed the narrative elsewhere of an approach followed by a 'maverick', an 'outlier', an 'outrider', and one that should not be emulated. On the BBC – in a country where the death toll just over a month later would top 100,000 and continue rising – the king's words had been accompanied by the figures of the high death rate in Sweden.[27] Deflection technique? The UK had handled things just so much better!

Could the Opposition Have Done Better? – Would There be Resignations?

Could the centre-right have done things differently?

There had not been much sign of that, indeed from the start of the crisis until the summer, the opposition parties had been right behind Löfven. In April, when it was already apparent that the Swedish death rate was far higher than in neighbouring countries, Busch, the Christian Democrat leader, had referred to him as her 'commander-in-chief'.[28] In June, in an interview with *Expressen*, she had said that if she had been prime minister, she might have chosen the same path as the government.[29]

Earlier, in a YouTube speech to the nation in March, Åkesson, the Sweden Democrat leader, had also placed himself firmly behind the prime minister. 'Stefan Löfven', he declared, 'you are not alone in this', we face coronavirus 'as a united country'.[30]

Then there was Kristersson, leader of the Moderates, probably the most constructive and strongest among the opposition leaders. However, while happy to criticise the government for not being fast enough on testing, contact-tracing, infection tracking, isolation, and PPE, he seemed less critical of Moderate-led regions that had chosen to ignore the building up of emergency stocks of PPE which had been their responsibility. Kristersson had been quick enough to accuse the government of hiding behind the public health agency and other authorities, but blame could be laid at the door of the Moderates too. At national level, he as leader of the party was holding Social Democratic ministers to account, and they in turn were holding regional councils led by the Moderates to account, and they in turn were simply shrugging their shoulders.[31] So, just who was going to fall on his or her sword? Was anyone going to resign over the failure?

From the Moderates came a demand for the resignation of Hallengren, the health and social affairs minister. Writing in *Expressen*, Matilda Ekeblad, chair of the Moderate Youth League (*Moderata ungdomsförbundet, MUF*) said that it would be fitting if the government took responsibility. 'A total failure. Hallengren should go!' screamed the headline. Throughout the year, the country had heard the regions calling for leadership from the government, and the government then passing the buck to agencies, boards, local authorities, and back to the regions again. When something positive happened, government ministers had been quick to take the credit, but when there was a setback, the fault lay elsewhere.[32]

Responsibility rested with the highest politicians in the land, said Ekeblad, and those holding a ministerial role, also held ministerial responsibility. Hallengren should shoulder the responsibilities that came with her job. Why, for example, had the municipalities been so unprepared for the rapid spread of infection across the country – a spread that had led to the deaths of so many of the elderly? Why had there been no prioritization of emergency preparedness? Why had neither the government nor Hallengren in particular, reacted or acted? Getting the vaccine programme underway, which was a positive, did not mean that the government could escape its responsibility for what had happened before that, the negative.[33]

Löfven's ministers had ducked and dived, but could no longer escape responsibility, and it was now time for Hallengren to resign. Tardiness and lack of leadership had led to the miserable failure of the Swedish strategy, and the health and social affairs minister had not lived up to the expectations of the post.[34]

Daniel Suhonen, co-founder of the Reformists movement within the Social Democrats, and director of the think tank Katalyst, suggested that the prime minister might have to end up sacking Hallengren. If Sweden had escaped the second wave of coronavirus, and what had amounted to a lockdown, then the strategy would have been judged successful, Suhonen claimed in a report by *Svenska Dagbladet*. However, with so many sick and so many deaths, it had clearly been a failure.[35]

Could any of the blame be placed elsewhere? Maybe on the Swedish 'government model' itself – *den svenska förvaltningsmodellen* – the convention of delegating responsibility to whichever powerful agency was responsible for the day-to-day running of their sector. In terms of the strategy to fight the pandemic, the delegated agency was Tegnell's and Carlson's public health agency.

Gro Harlem Brundtland, former Norwegian prime minister, and former head of the WHO was reported to have said in *VG* (the tabloid newspaper *Verdens Gang*), that it was 'completely unbelievable' that the public health agency had been in control for so long, and it was surprising that the government had followed agency assessments. I had watched it develop, shaken my head, and asked how was that possible? How Tegnell had judged the situation was one thing, but Sweden was a country with a government and parliament.[36]

So, what had government and parliamentarians been doing? Would anyone resign? Or would it take until the 2022 General Election before there was any reckoning? Perhaps that reckoning would come after the first reporting of the Corona Commission.

New Parliamentary Session, 2020–21 – A COVID-19 Budget

The prime ministerial statement given by Löfven at the opening of the new parliamentary session on 8 September 2020 had not been short on references to COVID-19.

COVID-19 was 'testing' the country and would shape the country 'for a long time to come'. Society was equipped to deal with new outbreaks, he said, and the government had decided to take part in the EU joint procurement of vaccines. Large-scale testing, physical distancing, and contact-tracing would continue. COVID-19 would be managed by Swedes together, and together they would work the country out of the crisis and build it better. Sweden had been given the chance 'to simultaneously create jobs and address societal changes', and this would be done by investing in healthcare, care of older people and in climate transition.[37]

COVID-19 had severely impacted people's lives and health, but the economy had also been hit. When the virus had arrived in Sweden, the country's national debt had been at its lowest since 1977, and this economic strength enabled all the mitigation measures that had been put in place, saving jobs and businesses. To move forward, transmission rates would still have to be kept low, but the transition from crisis-response policies to long-term investment was beginning. The budget bill – an historic budget bill – would contain new proposals worth more than SEK 100 billion.[38] Additionally, during the pandemic crisis the finance minister, Magdalena Andersson, had presented fifteen supplementary budgets and thanks to good government finances, it had been possible to meet the cost of the measures. Prior to the pandemic, the Swedish national debt had been around 35 per cent of GDP, and after the pandemic it was just under 40 per cent. The average in the EU was just over 70 per cent. Sweden's situation was a strong one, offering opportunity to ride out the crisis.[39]

Additionally, the Swedish economy was very open and export dependent, and so when the world suffered, so did Sweden. However, Sweden's economy had done much better than comparable countries. The world economy was

2.9 per cent smaller after 2021 than it would have been according to an OECD forecast before the pandemic: the Eurozone was 2.1 per cent smaller, and the US economy was 1.2 per cent smaller. But Sweden's economy was 0.4 per cent bigger – which was even more exceptional given that the government introduced much less fiscal stimulus than most other countries.[40]

COVID-19 had brought many people their first experience of working from home – to those who were able to – with remote working and digital meetings becoming the norm. To meet this demand, the expansion of digital infrastructure would continue. It had to be possible to live and work anywhere in the country, and opportunities for operating a business in rural areas would continue to be improved. Investment in housing and infrastructure was an effective way of stimulating the economy on the one hand and creating job opportunities on the other. The government intended to present an infrastructure bill to the *Riksdag* in the coming year, containing proposals for the long-term development of Swedish infrastructure. Currently, the government was making the biggest rail investment of modern times.[41]

COVID-19 had exposed the weak points in Swedish society, not least in the care of the elderly, and these could only be mended through substantial investment. Those working in care for older people had an important job involving great responsibility, and the work had to be attractive and receive clear recognition. A care for older people initiative was to be implemented to increase skill levels, allowing personnel – often on insecure contracts and working in several care homes at once – to train as nursing assistants or licenced practical nurses during paid working hours. This would lead to more than 10,000 new permanent jobs in the sector.[42]

In his statement, Löfven referred to the solidarity that had characterised Sweden during the crisis. This would be needed in the future too, for the task of strengthening the country was a joint one involving social partners, civil society, and the engagement of individuals.[43]

Inquiry Into Constitutional Preparedness for Future Pandemics – Report

In September 2021, the government had appointed a commission of inquiry with the task of reviewing the Communicable Diseases Control Act and updating the legislation. Headed by Lars Hedengran, the inquiry would take as its starting point the measures that had been implemented during the COVID-19 pandemic. Work of the inquiry on extraordinary infection control measures were to be reported on no later than 31 August 2023.

Published on 19 September 2023, the final report, 'Some infectious disease control issues within social services and social insurance' / 'Några smittskyddsfrågor inom socialtjänsten och socialförsäkringen' (SOU 2023:56) had proposed that individuals requiring extensive care needs, and who were perhaps unable to protect themselves from infection, might be moved without their consent to a safer environment in order to prevent the spread of infection, and to receive equivalent care and support. For relocation to be made, the individual must either be, or be presumed to be, infected with a disease that is dangerous to society, and through their behaviour, risk infecting other residents.[44]

A couple of months earlier, the Standing Committee on the Constitution (*KU*) had presented its report.

KU Reports on Its Investigation of Sweden's Handling of the Pandemic

The question of how the government had handled the COVID-19 pandemic as it gripped Sweden had always been in the background.

Tasked year by year to review government action on important issues and to examine the performance of ministers including the prime minister, the parliamentary Standing Committee on the Constitution had been questioning ministers, agency directors, and others, on the actions they had taken to deal with coronavirus. This powerful parliamentary committee, headed by Enström, reported in June 2021, identifying a number of areas in which the government had fallen short of its obligations.

The committee had found that there was a lack of clarity in who was responsible for testing and contact-tracing. These could have been speeded up in spring 2020 if the government had acted sooner to ensure regional authorities had sufficient funds to do that. In addition, the government ought to have ordered the public health agency to develop a national strategy to expand testing and contact-tracing sooner.[45]

There had also been a lack of clarity in who had been charged with purchasing PPE and other equipment for local and regional authorities. Additionally, several suppliers had believed that they could only sell equipment to the board of health and welfare.[46]

The committee also criticized the government for not putting forward sooner its proposals for a Pandemic Law (*Pandemilag*) and its more extensive powers. The Pandemic Law had been rushed through only in January 2021. Contradicting itself somewhat, the committee argued that parliament should have been allowed more time for the new bill to be processed.[47]

Additionally, the government's decision to cap the number of people allowed to attend public gatherings and events, had constituted a significant restriction on constitutionally protected rights and freedoms. At an earlier stage, the government should have tasked the public health agency to review continuously the epidemiological necessity of such limits.[48]

While criticism had been directed at the government generally, Enström had picked out a few individuals in particular: Löfven, the prime minister; Hallengren, the minister of social affairs; and Damberg, the interior minister. It would have been desirable for government strategy to have been documented to a greater degree than it had been, Enström had said. If there were going to be a strategy, it should have been well-anchored and well-prepared, but the committee found that it hadn't been.[49]

After the report had been published, Åkesson again accused the government of hiding behind agencies and authorities to a great extent. Crisis preparedness should have been much better. 'The government chose to turn a deaf ear' with tragic consequences. Over 14,000 dead and over 1,000,000 people infected was 'one of the great betrayals of our time', he had written.[50]

Hallengren recognized that there had been 'a number of shortcomings', and it was clear that what the committee had said, not least on the constitutional matter, was important and would require clarification or legislation in anticipation of future crises.[51]

On the delay to testing and contract-tracing in early-2020, she said that roles, responsibilities, money, and principles had all been clarified in an agreement with the municipalities and regions (with *Sveriges Kommuner och Regioner, SKR*), but with hindsight that could have been reached earlier. As for Swedish crisis preparedness and management, the government met the pandemic with the existing constitution, with municipal self-government, and with the principle of responsibility. Any grey border areas between state, municipalities and regions would have to be identified and assessed.[52]

After the dust had settled around the *KU* report, the second interim report of the Corona Commission, appointed in June 2020, and headed by Mats Melin, was awaited. It was expected in autumn 2021.

Second Interim Report – *Coronakommissionen*

By autumn 2021, prime minister Stefan Löfven had gone. In late-June, he had resigned after losing a confidence vote in parliament, the first Swedish prime minister to fall in this way, and not over the COVID-19 strategy, or even migration policy, but over market rents. Although he was back leading another minority government a few days later in early-July, a month later he announced that he would be stepping down. In November he was replaced by his colleague, former finance minister Magdalena Andersson.

Though Löfven had gone, COVID-19 remained, plaguing the world in a third pandemic year, and Melin's Corona Commission was still investigating and carrying out its task. The first interim report of the commission had come out on 7 December 2020, and the second had been presented at a press conference on 29 October 2021 just as delegates were preparing to travel to Gothenburg for the Social Democratic Party congress. The focus of the report was 'Sweden during the pandemic', and it was presented in two volumes, *Infection and infection control*, and *Healthcare and public health*.

The report concluded that the response to the pandemic had been slow and described initial measures to control the virus as insufficient to stop or sharply limit the spread of the virus. In spring 2020, the Swedish measures had come late, not only compared with the neighbouring Nordic countries but also in relation to the spread of infection prevailing in Sweden. It had also been far too slow in building up enough testing capacity and the commission believed this to be partly because of a lack of resources, partly because of a lack of preparedness, and partly because testing on the necessary scale had never taken place before. The commission placed the responsibility for testing on the regions, and the report described as a 'car crash' a dispute arising over funding and liability, and which contributed to the delay in implementing large-scale testing until after the first wave of the pandemic. Scaling up of testing had gone significantly slower in Sweden than in Norway, Denmark, and Finland.[53]

The choice of measures early in the pandemic had been crucial in the development of the spread of infection across the country and when coronavirus arrived it had spread quickly, mainly from travellers returning from winter sports resorts in Austria. Because of limited testing, Sweden could not get enough of a picture of how many positive cases there had been in the early stages of the spread. Instead, the number of hospital admissions and the death rate were given as a description of the situation despite these reflecting a later stage in the development of the disease and thus offering a delayed picture of the spread of infection. If it had been hospital admissions and the death rate that dominated in Swedish surveillance of the pandemic there was every chance that this was one of the reasons for the lateness characterising the country's pandemic management.[54]

When subsequent waves of the virus had emerged, Sweden had brought in more substantial measures, but this had not happened because of any new science. The report found that the introduction of restrictions that had been explicitly avoided during the first wave created reasonable confusion among the population and may have contributed to poorer compliance.[55]

The report also found that Sweden's emergency stockpile had been dismantled over several years and at the start of the outbreak it had been in effect non-existent. The 'just-in-time' management strategy meant that stocks had been kept as small and as efficient as possible. The resulting shortage of personal protective equipment (PPE) had become so acute in spring 2020 that staff occasionally had to work without adequate equipment. Several weeks in over February and early-March had been wasted before the government commissioned the relevant authority to secure access to PPE.[56]

Some positives could be found in the report. Infectious disease and intensive care units had largely managed the transition to pandemic care, and in general COVID-19 patients had received the care they needed. This had been achieved despite the lack of pandemic planning and the provision of extra capacity. Indeed, in dealing with the pandemic, healthcare had stretched existing staff to breaking point.[57]

Despite the many shortcomings identified by the commission, the report found that as far as comparison with Europe was concerned, Sweden appeared to be average in terms of the number of deaths during the first and second waves of the pandemic. During the third wave, the death toll had been low, and Sweden had done better than most countries in Europe.[58]

Who Would be Held Accountable?

The second interim report had come out just as Löfven was stepping down from his role as prime minister. Johan Carlson, director-general of the public health agency was also retiring, and at 65-years old, the state epidemiologist, Anders Tegnell, was likely to be leaving post quite soon too. So, who was going to be held accountable for the failings identified?

Would the first, second, and final report, or indeed the pandemic still be talking points once the election came round? If they were, would anyone notice that most of the opposition had supported the government's measures at the time – or the initial measures at least?

In the absence of Löfven, Carlson, and Tegnell, would Lena Hallengren, the health minister, take the blame for the failings identified in the second report? Would she take the blame for failings expected to be listed in the final report in February 2022? Would she be found a role in Andersson's new government? And would Andersson herself have anything to answer to, or would her cabinet position looking after the country's finances during the pandemic allow her sufficient distance from the health crisis to avoid harsh criticism or to make her vulnerable? (Later on, Löfven had written that at the height of the pandemic, Hallengren notified him that she had breast cancer, but that with a treatment plan in place she intended to work on as usual, but more from home in Kalmar where she was having her treatment[59]).

The second interim report had been harsh, but it was easy for the government to evade responsibility because the failings of so many other 'accomplices' had been highlighted. The government, it seemed, had not seen any reason for self-criticism over the coronavirus crisis. During an interview for *Dagens Nyheter* in September, Hallengren had said that it looked as if Sweden had 'come out of this rather well', nor could she think of anything specific that she had regretted during the crisis. Indeed, Löfven had also said the same in October, indicating that there was nothing that he would have done differently while prime minister.[60]

Sweden's strategy had its critics from the very start, many of them advocating a more robust approach, and for their trouble they were sometimes treated like traitors in an environment in which patriotism had prevailed in defence of, and in identification with, the different choice that Sweden had taken. There had been huge public support for the strategy and confidence in the public health agency had been high, and the prime minister too had received a sharp boost in the polls. Even the opposition had been behind the government with none of the opposition parties putting forward an alternative strategy during the all-important months of February and March 2020. Jimmie Åkesson would not be allowed to forget his 'emotional' words in a speech to the nation on YouTube in March 2020: 'Stefan Löfven, you are not alone in this', we face coronavirus 'as a united country'.[61]

Of course, there were at least two important reasons why the opposition had given their support to Löfven. One was that public opinion had also done so. The other was that many of the municipalities and regions were controlled by opposition parties, and much of crisis management had been in the hands of local and regional government.[62]

The final report of Melin's Corona Commission expected in February 2022 was eagerly anticipated.

Final Report – *Coronakommissionen*

On 25 February 2022, the final report had been duly published, but it had made its appearance the day after Vladimir Putin's invasion of Ukraine – an unprecedented assault on European security – and it would be partially buried by that event.

The opening statement of the summary to the Melin Commission report had been a positive one. 'In comparison with the rest of Europe', it began, Sweden had 'come through the pandemic relatively well'. It was 'among the countries with the lowest excess mortality over the period 2020–21'. In comparison to the first and second interim reports which had been sharply critical, the final report had given unexpectedly strong support for the Swedish approach.[63]

The report had concluded that Sweden's path had the significant benefit that people had 'not been forced to the same extent as in many other countries to comply with regulations restricting their personal freedom'. The strategy and its 'focus on rapid and vigorous monetary and fiscal policy interventions' had been the correct one 'in the area of economic crisis management'. In terms of disease prevention and control, focus 'on advice and recommendations which people were expected to follow voluntarily', had been 'fundamentally correct', and 'meant that citizens retained more of their personal freedom than in many other countries'. When compared to the approach to disease prevention and control taken elsewhere, in the view of the commission, the Swedish strategy differed 'less in its description of the overarching aim than in the measures used to achieve that aim'.[64]

Nevertheless, the report did contain criticisms of the way in which the strategy had been implemented. The commission found that 'measures taken were too few and should have come sooner'. The report stated that in February/March 2020 intrusive disease prevention and control measures should have been 'more rigorous', and that it was 'remarkable' that the limit of fifty for public gatherings did not come until 29 March. In the absence of a plan to protect the elderly and vulnerable, 'earlier and additional steps should have been taken to try to slow community transmission'. Additionally, those spending winter sports holidays in Italy, February/March 'should have been provided with clearer instructions to home-quarantine' on their return. A 'temporary ban on entry to Sweden should have been introduced no later than mid-March' as in Denmark and Norway, resulting in a common Nordic approach – something that was never achieved. On face-coverings, the commission considered that after a shortage of masks had been remedied, the public health agency ought to have recommended their use in indoor settings and on public transport, rather than dismissing their use. On the other hand, the commission believed 'that the right balance was struck in keeping preschools and compulsory schools open'.[65] Studies had shown this in relation to learning loss.

Of importance for the future was the question of learning loss when students were not allowed to go to school for months on end. On average, students across the world lost out on more than one third of a normal year's worth of learning. Closures had hit poorer families harder as they could not compensate from school closure in the way that socio-economically advantaged families could. In the USA, the Department of Education concluded that half of American students began 2023 a full year behind grade level in at least one subject (grade level is a level of study completed by a student in any given year). In sharp contrast, Swedish elementary scholars suffered no learning loss during the pandemic.[66]

The commission report was also critical of the government's crisis management and lack of clarity in handling disease prevention and control, essentially allowing the public health agency to set the pace. The government had a too one-sided dependence on assessments made by the agency, and that these assessments ultimately rested on a single person – the director-general, Carlson. This was 'not a satisfactory arrangement' for decision-making during a crisis. The commission believed that the government ought to 'have assumed leadership of all aspects of crisis management from the outset' and 'should also have assumed clearer leadership of overall communication with the public'. The government ought to 'have been able to overcome obstacles to clear national leadership' such as the degree of autonomy traditionally possessed by government agencies.[67]

In addition, the report highlighted class differences in the impact of the pandemic on people. The commission found that the measures introduced had 'often been better suited to a well-educated middle class, well placed to protect themselves from infection, navigate the health care system and work from home'. Secondly, groups already disadvantaged had been hardest hit by COVID-19 in terms of severe illness and death. Thirdly, working from home was easier for those not living in overcrowded housing, and fourthly, people in a range of occupations – in health and social care, services, and education – were obviously unable to perform their duties at home.[68]

Although Sweden had come through the pandemic relatively well, recording some of the lowest excess mortality in Europe, 2020–21, the commission observed that 'to learn lessons we must not forget what the situation looked like in the spring of 2020'.[69]

Where Did the Blame Lie? What Did the Commission Recommend?

The commission found that the slow Swedish response to the pandemic had come because the public health agency 'adopted a position informed by a demand for evidence – rather than a precautionary approach – and had a defensive view of the prospects of slowing the spread of the virus'. This resulted in it introducing and advocating 'limited, late and not very vigorous measures'. Responsibility had rested on the director-general – Carlson.[70]

The commission also found that the government, and Löfven, were 'responsible for having accepted largely uncritically, right up to the late autumn of 2020, the assessments of its expert agency'. The prime minister had also failed 'to issue directives' calling for the agency to change course.[71] The commission had observed that the government had been too passive, relying on and listening too much to the public health agency – sitting on its lap, as it were – instead of being clearer themselves on matters. In his autobiography, Löfven wrote that before the government made a decision, they would 'of course always listen to the public health agency and other expert authorities. It would be strange otherwise, and yet this was what had been held against us, later'.[72]

The aim of the commission had been to consider how management of the next crisis affecting health and society could be improved, and it did have recommendations to make. It recommended 'far-reaching administrative reform' which should 'be made the subject of new, open-minded deliberations' as soon as possible. It called for the establishment of a 'body providing clear national crisis leadership' reporting directly to the government. During serious societal crises, this body would 'obtain information from all relevant stakeholders, lay down clear guidelines for their work' and 'issue binding directives to public authorities'. In the Swedish crisis management system, the basic principle ought to be that, in a threatening situation 'decision-makers should not passively wait for a better understanding but actively take steps to counter the threat'. This meant that it was 'better to act than wait for better data for decision-making'. The commission called for a cross-party committee of inquiry to consider changes to both the principles and the organisation of crisis management. It also recommended the re-organisation of the disease prevention and control framework so that the public health agency no longer had sole responsibility for providing the government with decision support data on the issues involved in fighting a pandemic.[73]

While the criticisms of the commission had been sharp and precise – and balanced with some positivity – it was hard to believe that questions over pandemic management would become an election issue, despite all the sound and fury after the first interim report, and to a lesser degree after the second. In the first place, Löfven and Carlson had already gone, and Löfven's successor Andersson, who was finance minister at the time, had been highly praised by the commission. Then there was the matter of voter trust in, and support of, Tegnell the state epidemiologist, and the strategy of allowing the public health agency to take the lead in the crisis. Both the Social Democrats and the prime minister had been given high confidence ratings from voters, and Tegnell became a public celebrity, if not idol, even abroad. Finally, where had the opposition been during the early stages of the crisis? None of the opposition parties had demanded any stricter infection control measures during the vital months February/March 2020. 'You are not alone in this', Åkesson had declared in his support of Löfven. In addition, many of Sweden's regions – also criticised by the commission – were under the control of opposition parties. It had been the regions that were responsible for poor preparedness when the crisis emerged, and failures in testing and contact-tracing during the first wave of infections.[74]

The Final Chapter reflects on the Sweden that had emerged from the COVID-19 experience. Could it still be described as the 'outlier', the 'outrider', as Sweden the 'foolhardy'? How had it fared in comparison to other countries of comparable size? What became of the key players in the Swedish drama? Were there any loose ends to tie up? What became of the international pandemic treaty, and COVAX? And what about death statistics globally and nationally into 2025?

Notes

[1] Ahlander, Johan. and Simon Johnson, 'Sweden should have done more against coronavirus but broad strategy right: chief epidemiologist', *Reuters*, 3 June 2020, <https://www.reuters.com/articles/us-health-coronavirus-sweden-tegenll-idUSKBN23A15O> accessed 13 September 2020.

[2] Ibid.

[3] 'Mats Melin to chair COVID-19 inquiry in Sweden', Ministry of Health and Social Affairs, Government Offices of Sweden, 1 July 2020, <https://www.government.se/press-releases/2020/06/mats-melin-to-chair-covid-19-inquiry-in-sweden/> and, Committee terms of reference. Summary. Dir. 2020:74. Evaluation of the measures to tackle the outbreak of the virus that causes the disease COVID-19. Decision made at the Cabinet meeting on 30 June 2020, p. 1. Socialdepartementet, Regeringen / Government Offices of Sweden.

[4] Ministry of Health and Social Affairs, 1 July 2020, as note 3.

[5] Ibid.

[6] Ibid.

[7] 'Swedish healthcare watchdog condemns serious flaws in elderly care during pandemic', *The Local*, 24 November 2020, <https://www.thelocal.se/20201124/swedish-healthcare-watchdog-condemns-serious-flaws-in-elderly-care-during-pandemic> accessed 10 December 2020.

[8] 'What does the first report from Sweden's coronavirus commission tell us?' *The Local*, 15 December 2020, <https://www.thelocal.se/20201215/what-does-the-first-report-from-swedens-coronavirus-commission-tell-us> accessed 29 January 2021, and, 'Äldreomsorgen under pandemin'. Delbetänkande av Coronakommissionen, English Summary, Statens Offentliga Utredningar SOU 2020:80, Stockholm, 7 December 2020, p. 2, p. 8, p. 11 <https://coronakommissionen.com/wp-content/uploads/2020/12/summary.pdf> accessed 31 October 2021.

[9] Ibid., Statens Offentliga Utredningar, p. 2, p. 9.

[10] Ibid., p. 1, p. 2, p. 9, p. 10.

[11] Ibid., p. 1, p. 5, p. 8, p. 9.

[12] Ibid., p. 3, p. 8, p. 11.

[13] Löfven, Stefan. i samarbete med Ulrika Knutson. *Svetsare och statsminister*, p. 180, p. 181, p. 189.

[14] Duxbury, Charlie. 'How Sweden's prime minister plans to save his career from coronavirus' Politico.eu, 24 December 2020, <https://www.politico.eu/article/stefan-lofven-sweden-coronavirus-escape/> accessed 31 October 2021.

[15] Ibid.

[16] Ibid.

[17] 'Explained: What can the parliament's inquiry tell us about Sweden's coronavirus strategy?' *The Local*, 26 March 2021, <https://www.thelocal.se/20210326/explained-ku-what-can-the-parliaments-inquiry-tell-us-about-swedens-coronavirus-strategy/> accessed 27 March 2021.

[18] Ibid.

[19] Delin, Michael. and Hanna Jakobson. 'Dan Eliasson i KU: MSB ville larma tidigare', *Dagens Nyheter*, 26 March 2021, <https://www.dn.se/sverige/dan-eliasson-i-ku-msb-ville-larma-tidigare/> and, 'Sweden's crisis agency wanted earlier and more Covid measures, claims former director', *The Local*, 26 March 2021, <https://www.thelocal.se/20210326/swedens-crisis-agency-wanted-earlier-and-more-covid-measures-claims-former-director/> accessed 27 March 2021.

[20] Ibid., *The Local*, 26 March 2021.

21 Stenberg, Ewa. 'Därför har väljarna inte get Löfven skulden', *Dagens Nyheter*, 27 April 2021, <https://www.dn.se/sverige/ewa-stenberg-darfor-har-valjarna-inte-gett-lofven-skulden/> accessed 28 April 2021.

22 Ibid.

23 'King of Sweden on the coronavirus pandemic: We have failed', *The Local*, 17 December 2020, <https://www.thelocal.se/20201217/king-of-sweden-on-the-coronavirus-pandemic-we-have-failed> and, 'Kungens pandemikritik ger eko i världen', *Dagens Nyheter*, 17 December 2020, <https://www.dn.se/sverige/kungen-om-pandemin-vi-har-misslyckats/> accessed 30 January 2021.

24 Ibid., both articles.

25 Ibid.

26 *Dagens Nyheter*, 17 December 2020, as note 23.

27 Ibid.

28 Franke, Peter. 'Se dig själv i spegeln, Ebba',*VF (Värmlands Folkblad)*, 8 June 2020, <https://www.vf.se/2020/06/08/se-dig-sjalv-i-spegeln-ebba/> accessed 3 February 2021.

29 Sokolnicki, Amanda. 'Moderaternas roll i pandemin är ingenting att vara stolt över', *Dagens Nyheter*, 19 December 2020, <https://www.dn.se/ledare/amanda-sokolnicki-moderaternas-roll-i-pandemin-ar-ingenting-att-vara-stolt-over/> accessed 3 February 2021.

30 Ibid. The YouTube speech referred to was, Åkesson, J. 'Jimmie Åkessons tal till nationen'. YouTube. 26 March 2020, <https://www.youtube.com/watch?v=d1ZqwLzRBQk> accessed 2 November 2021.

31 Ibid.

32 Ekeblad, Matilda. Förbundsordförande MUF, 'Misslyckandet är totalt – avgå, Lena Hallengren', *Expressen*, 20 December 2020, <https://www.expressen.se/debatt/misslyckandet-ar-totalt-avga-lena-hallengren/> accessed 2 February 2021.

33 Ibid.

34 Ibid.

35 Treijs, Erica. and Eric Olsson. 'Suhonen: Kanske måste Löfven offra Hallengren', *Svenska Dagbladet*, 20 December 2020, <https://www.svd.se/suhonen-kanske-maste-lofven-offra-hallengren> accessed 2 February 2021.

36 Muri, Karin. and Janne Møller-Hansen. 'Må bare si fra', *VG* (*Verdens Gang*), 20 December 2020, <https://www.vg.no/forbruker/helse/i/jBvGk9/maa-bare-si-fra> accessed 2 February 2021.

37 Statement of Government Policy given by Prime Minister Stefan Löfven before the Riksdag, Government Offices of Sweden, 8 September 2020, pp.1–2.

38 Ibid., p. 3.

39 Löfven, as note 13, p. 185.

40 Norberg, Johan. 'Sweden during the pandemic. Pariah or paragon?' p. 9, *CATO policy analysis*, No. 959, 29 August 2023, Cato Institute, <https://www.cato.org/sites/cato.org/files/2023-08/policy-analysis-959-no-link.pdf> accessed 6 February 2025.

41 Statement of Government Policy, as note 37, pp. 4–5.

42 Ibid., pp.6–7.

43 Ibid., p. 2.

44 Några smittskyddsfrågor inom socialtjänsten och socialförsäkringen, SOU 2023:56, Press release from the Ministry of Health, Government Office of Sweden, 19 September 2023, <https://www.regeringen.se/rattsliga-dokument/statens-offentliga-utredningar/2023/09/sou-202356/> accessed 16 January 2025.

45 'KU:s granskning av regeringen är klar', Aktuellt, Sveriges Riskdag, 3 June 2021, <https://www.riksdagen.se/sv/aktuellt/2021/jun/3/kusgranskning-av-regeringen-ar-klar/> accessed 7 June 2021.

46 Ibid.

47 Ibid.

48 Ibid.

49 Jakobson, Hanna. and Amanda Dahl. 'KU: Regeringen har brustit i hanteringen av pandemin', *Dagens Nyheter*, 3 June 2021, <https://www.dn.se/sverige/ku-regeringen-har-brustit-i-hanteringen-av-pandemin/> accessed 6 June 2021.

50 Ibid.

51 Ibid.

52 Ibid.

53 Dahl, Amanda. 'Skarp kritik mot svensk coronahantering: Otillräckliga åtgärder', *Dagens Nyheter*, 29 October 2021, <https://www.dn.se/sverige/skarp-kritik-mot-svensk-coronahantering-otillrackliga-atgarder/> and, 'Sverige under pandemin'. Volym 1 'Smittspridning och smittskydd'. Volym 2 'Sjukvård och folkhälsa'. Delbetänkande 2 / Interim Report 2. Coronakommissionen, Summary in English. Statens Offentliga Utredningar SOU 2021:89, Stockholm, 29 October 2021, p. 1, p. 2, p. 6, p. 8–9, <https://coronakommissionen.co/wp-content/uploads/2021/10/summary-sweden-in-the-pandemic.pdf> accessed 29 October 2021.

54 Ibid., Interim Report 2, p.3, p. 4, p. 5, p.6.

55 Ibid., p. 7.

56 Ibid., p. 12. p. 22, p.23.

57 Ibid., p. 14, p. 15.

58 Ibid., p. 1.

59 Löfven, as note 13, pp. 176–7.

60 Stenberg, Ewa. 'Hallengren har en del att ångra – trots allt', *Dagens Nyheter*, 30 October 2021, <https://dn.se/sverige/ewa-stenberg-hallengren-har-en-del-att-angra-trots-allt/> accessed 31 October 2021. In her piece, Stenberg refers to an article by Hans Olsson, 'Hallengren: Sverige har kommit väl ut ur detta', *Dagens Nyheter*, 28 September 2021, <https://www.dn.se/sverige/hallengren-sverige-har-kommit-val-ut-ur-detta/> accessed 31 October 2021.

61 Ibid., Stenberg. Stenberg had reported Åkesson's words in April 2020, in the article 'Än så länge politisk enighet om den liberala coronastrategin', *Dagens Nyheter*, <https://www.dn.se/nyheter/sverige/ewa-stenberg-an-sa-lange-politisk-enighet-om-den-liberala-coronastrategin/> as had her DN colleague, Amanda Sokolnicki, in 'Moderaternas roll i pandemin är ingenting att vara stolt över', *Dagens Nyheter*, 19 December 2020, <https://www.dn.se/ledare/amanda-sokolnicki-moderaternas-roll-i-pandemin-ar-ingenting-att-vara-stolt-over/> accessed 2 November 2021. The YouTube speech referred to was, Åkesson, J. 'Jimmie Åkessons tal till nationen'. YouTube. 26 March 2020, <https://www.youtube.com/watch?v=d1ZqwLzRBQk> accessed 2 November 2021.

62 Ibid., Stenberg, 30 October 2021.

63 'Sverige under pandemin'. Volym 1 'Samhällets, företagens och enskildas ekonomi'. Volym 2 'Förutsättningar, vägval och utvärdering'. Slutbetänkande av Coronakommissionen. Summary in English. Statens Offentliga Utredningar SOU 2022:10, Stockholm, 25 February 2022, p. 1, <https://coronakommission.com/wp-content/uploads/2022/02/summary_20220225.pdf> accessed 25 February 2022.

64 Ibid., p. 3, p. 7.

65 Ibid., p. 3, p. 8, p. 9, p. 10-11.

66 Norberg, as note 40.

67 'Sverige under pandemin', as note 63, p. 4, p. 13.

68 Ibid., p.2.

69 Ibid., p. 1.

70 Ibid., p. 18.

71 Ibid., p. 19.
72 Löfven, as note 13, pp. 177–8.
73 'Sverige under pandemin', as note 63, p. 3, p. 20, p. 25.
74 Stenberg, Ewa. 'Svårt att utkräva politiskt ansvar för dödsfallen', *Dagens Nyheter*, 25 February 2022, <https://www.dn.se/sverige/ewa-stenberg-svart-att-utkrava-politiskt-ansvar-for-dodsfallen/> accessed 26 February 2022.

Final Chapter

Foolhardy, Exceptional, or Just Principled?

In autumn 2021, Sweden's prime minister Stefan Löfven had stepped down. Earlier, in late-June, he had resigned after losing a confidence vote in parliament, and although he was back leading another minority government a few days later, he announced soon after that he was leaving the premiership and his role as leader of the Social Democrats. In November he was replaced in both roles by his colleague, former finance minister Magdalena Andersson.

Though Löfven had gone, COVID-19 remained, plaguing the world in a third pandemic year, 2022, and Melin's Corona Commission was still investigating and carrying out its task, reporting finally in February that year, an event buried by Putin's invasion of Ukraine.

Cumulatively since the start of the COVID-19 pandemic in Sweden and until end-December 2021, some 15,310 coronavirus deaths had occurred, and it was clear that the term in office of Sweden's 33rd prime minister would almost certainly be defined by these deaths, particularly the deaths of large numbers of elderly people in residential care, and by the almost 'hands-off' approach that his government had taken towards the crisis. COVID-19 and its aftermath had occupied the attention of the country and of his cabinet and government for just over one quarter of his tenure.

As has been seen, the Corona Commission found that Löfven's government was to blame for failures in the protection of the country's care home residents. Central government agencies did not have enough of an overview of the problems and deficiencies in municipal elderly care, and the government held overall responsibility for this. Responsibility also rested on previous governments that had possessed knowledge of the structural shortcomings in elderly care. Even so, the opening statement of the summary to Melin's Corona Commission report had been a positive one. 'In comparison with the rest of Europe', it began, Sweden had 'come through the pandemic relatively well'.

At the start of it all in early-2020, the Löfven government had enjoyed public confidence for its handling of COVID-19 with support for the sitting administration rising when the pandemic struck. Later, neither a run of political crises throughout 2021, nor the state of health and social care during the pandemic, nor even the war in Ukraine, had influenced the voting intention of Swedish voters during the 2022 General Election campaign. It had been crime, law and order, and energy, that had been at the top of the agenda. It had neither been the pandemic nor Ukraine that had been discussed the most, rather food prices, growing criminality, and the economy.[1]

For Löfven as a politician, and who had lost his foster-mother, Iris Melander aged 90,[2] during the pandemic, the worst thing was that it just 'never ended'. From the 'first anxious days' of early-2020 to his departure from office and as party leader in autumn 2021, every day 'was overshadowed by coronavirus'. Questions around it 'ground constantly inside us all the time'. There was the 'nagging worry, the harsh criticism, disagreement within medical science, vaccines and testing, comparison with other countries, social media, and accusations that we were killing the old'. It had been a completely new virus, and a completely new situation that had to be tackled, and no one knew how it would end.[3]

No longer in parliament, having stepped down from his Västernorrland constituency as well as his role as prime minister and party leader, Löfven successively took up an assignment with the UN, an appointment with SIPRI, presidency of the Party of European Socialists, and a residency fellowship at the Harvard Kennedy School, John F. Kennedy School of Government, Cambridge, Massachusetts. In collaboration with Ulrika Knutson, journalist, author, and columnist, Löfven's autobiography was published in September 2024, a chapter of which dealt with *pandemin*.

In November, Löfven had been replaced as leader of his party, and as prime minister, by Andersson. Despite steering Sweden through the pandemic crisis with her package of budgets and financial mitigation measures, and avoiding the accusations of blame falling on colleagues, her tenure as Sweden's first female prime minister, and the country's 34th prime minister, lasted less than a year. She was voted out of office in October 2022 after losing the general election in September to Ulf Kristersson of the centre-right, who became the 35th prime minister. A new role in opposition followed for Andersson as Social Democratic party leader. Sweden had known three prime ministers in just under a year.

Lena Hallengren, health and social affairs minister in Löfven and Andersson cabinets since 2019, and a minister in other roles since 2002, had managed to avoid sacking or having to resign in wake of the *Coronakommission* reports, but her ministerial role also ended in October 2022. For a brief period from 2020, Hallengren had been a member of the Global Leaders Group on Antimicrobial

Resistance, a joint effort of the FAO, UNEP, the WHO, and the WOAH. In opposition, she was the Social Democrat group leader in the *Riksdag*.

In October 2021, Johan Carlson, director-general of the public health agency (*Folkhälsomyndigheten*), had retired and in November he was replaced by Karin Tegmark Wisell. In 2024, she was appointed as Sweden's ambassador for global health at the foreign ministry. Her role would be to mobilize and strengthen Sweden's work on health issues globally, particularly in areas where there remained many challenges: increased microbial resistance, pandemic risk, climate change, wars and conflict, and how all of these affected health and well-being. Olivia Wigzell at the National Board of Health and Welfare (*Socialstyrelsen*) had taken over Tegmark Wisell's public health role.[4]

Carlson's colleague at the public health agency during the pandemic, the state epidemiologist, Anders Tegnell, had stood down from his role in March 2022, to be replaced by Anders Lindblom, a specialist in infectious diseases. This new state epidemiologist subsequently stepped down too, at the end of June 2022 (though he served on until a successor could take over). Tegnell meanwhile seemed set for a new role at the WHO to assist as a senior expert in the task of making COVID-19 vaccine available to those countries unable to buy their own vaccines.[5]

Argument would continue over whether Sweden's controversial COVID-19 strategy had been successful or not, with Tegnell himself standing by it, though admitting there had been 'obviously a potential for improvement' in what had been done. Were the country 'to encounter the same disease again, knowing what we know about it today', he thought that they 'would settle on doing something in between what Sweden did and what the rest of the world has done'. There was an issue with how countries counted deaths, he believed, saying that comparisons between countries 'were unfair' because some were 'not reporting the actual death rates', while Sweden was 'the best in the world in reporting the actual number of dead'.[6] There had been room for positive acknowledgement of the Swedish approach.

Relying largely on social distancing, good hygiene, and targeted measures that kept schools, restaurants, and shops open, Sweden had emerged from the first year of pandemic (2020) with a smaller increase in its overall mortality rate than most European countries. While such analysis of data could not be interpreted as evidence that countries need not lockdown during pandemic events, it did acknowledge that the overall Swedish stance had its merits.[7]

In a compilation made by Reuters, and based on Eurostat statistics, Sweden had 7.7 per cent excess mortality in whole year 2020 compared to the average for the preceding four years (2015–19). Spain and Belgium which had chosen strict lockdown measures experienced excess mortality of 18.1 per cent (Spain) and 16.2

per cent (Belgium). Nevertheless, Swedish excess mortality that year was worse than its neighbours, with Denmark registering 1.5 per cent, Finland 1 per cent, and Norway no excess mortality. Of course, in any comparison made between countries, other factors had to be taken into account, such as age structure of the population, life expectancy, general health, household sizes, and even travel hubs and transport organisation in cities.[8] In any case, the number of COVID-19 dead was never going to be as simple a statistic as it seemed. Some countries did not count deaths outside hospital. If patients died at home or in nursing homes, they were not automatically included in the data sets. In Sweden, authorities administering population registration (births, deaths, marriages) automatically checked the lists of people who were infected, so everyone who died and had tested positive for the virus was counted as a COVID-19 death, even if they died from a heart attack or a fall. So, in effect, Sweden reported many who died 'with' COVID-19, not 'of' COVID-19.[9] And, Tegnell had made that point.

The Eurostat/Reuters data had been confirmed by comparisons found by the UK Office for National Statistics (ONS) over a six-month period in 2020 (rather than whole year). In comparisons of cumulative excess mortality between European countries and regions between early-January 2020 to end-June 2020, the UK experienced 3.1 per cent excess mortality compared to the average for the preceding four years (2015–19). Bulgaria had the highest at 18.2 per cent above average, Poland 13.3 per cent, and Romania 12.2 per cent. Norway had the lowest with 4.1 per cent below average, Sweden 4 per cent, and Iceland 3.9 per cent.[10]

More widely, looking at actual numbers of excess deaths in Europe and beyond on 31 December 2020, cumulative deaths in the USA from all causes compared to projection based on previous years (excess mortality) was 1,410 deaths per million, and in Sweden 764 deaths per million. Russia showed 2,560 deaths per million, Bulgaria 2,331, Romania 1,773, Poland 1,594, UK 1,188, Hungary 1,110, South Africa 958, Brazil 904 deaths per million, Türkiye 780. On 31 December 2023, the USA showed 3,968 deaths per million on the same measure, and Sweden 1,910.[11]

For his part, Tegnell believed that the Eurostat/Reuters data (2020) had raised questions, saying that while total shutdowns 'may have had an effect in the short term', when looking throughout the pandemic in the longer term 'you become more and more doubtful' about lockdowns.[12]

Some years on from 2020 when the pandemic first swept across Europe, the individual experience, the national experience, the continent-wide experience, and the global experience remained of interest. Indeed, the UK COVID-19 Inquiry had been concerned to understand the response taken to the pandemic in Sweden, and Tegnell had been called upon to present a witness statement in October 2023, particularly concerning any views or assessments he may have set out to the UK prime minister or other individuals.[13]

Set up to examine the UK response to, and the impact of, the COVID-19 pandemic, and to produce a factual narrative account, the UK COVID-19 Inquiry had begun its public hearings in June 2023. The inquiry would identify lessons to be learned and inform the preparations for future pandemics across the UK. Chaired by Heather Hallet, public hearings of the COVID-19 inquiry were expected to continue into 2026. The pandemic had affected everyone in the UK, and in many instances, continued to have a lasting impact. The inquiry offered the opportunity to share the impact that COVID-19 had on people – each experience being unique.[14]

In his testimony, Tegnell answered that he had concerns about how Sweden had not managed to protect the elderly and other disadvantaged groups compared to the population at large. At no time had Sweden adopted a herd immunity strategy. Such a strategy 'does not really exist', he stated. When asked if the strategy and response to COVID-19 changed in Sweden during the progress of the pandemic, he answered that the 'basic strategy was maintained', but 'adapted over time'. Additionally, concerning impositions, Tegnell confirmed to the inquiry that: working from home had been 'used throughout the whole pandemic'; social distancing had been 'used throughout the pandemic'; self-isolation requirements had been 'used throughout the pandemic but they were not mandatory'; and the use of face-coverings was 'only in buses and trains for a short time in early 2021'.[15] September 2023, Tegnell had also discussed with the chair of the Scottish COVID-19 Inquiry, the Swedish approach to developing and implementing a response to the pandemic.[16]

On herd immunity, Tegnell's critics might have disagreed. Hadn't public health authorities in Sweden relied on 'natural' herd immunity to be achieved through unchecked infection? Hadn't they 'ignored the science as it developed' and had 'deliberately failed to implement most useful preventive strategies?'[17]

The levels of autonomy and power enjoyed by public health authorities also excited criticism. They had 'preened themselves in the unexpected glow of attention' they had been given. At the same time, politicians in 'a weak coalition government' – Löfven's – had used as a fig leaf the supposed autonomy of the Swedish administrative system 'to abdicate responsibility for taking the reins'. No one had dared to call out the authorities in their bubble.[18] The opposition in the *Riksdag* wasn't off the hook either. In the earliest weeks, the political opposition had offered little opposition to the government.

In 2025, five years on from the first confirmed coronavirus case in Jönköping in late-January 2020, the first death on 11 March 2020 in Stockholm, and the full impact of the pandemic, it had been a moment for reflection, especially on the elderly in residential care who should have been protected but had died unnecessarily. In February 2025, Jakob Forssmed, the centre-right Christian Democrat minister for social affairs and public health in Kristersson's government, had referred to the loss suffered by so many in Sweden, and to the long-term health issues that remained. In these five years, society had 'undergone a comprehensive crisis' but had 'long since returned to normality', though COVID-19 had 'left lasting scars in the form of grief and loss'.[19]

He talked of the important measures taken within the public health agency to build 'a stronger system for surveillance of communicable diseases' which included 'increased epidemiological and microbiological surveillance'. Today, Sweden's capacity to manage a pandemic was better than in 2020, and a lesson learned was that such an event required 'clear political responsibility'.[20]

'Government governs the state in times of crisis', he continued, and that responsibility could not be handed over to public authorities. Crisis management required more than preparedness in the form of regulation or regulatory frameworks – rules, standards, guidelines – but rather it required the ability to act in a new set of circumstances in which, by definition, all the answers would not yet be apparent. There was a requirement to act proactively and decisively in both peacetime crises and in times of war or threat of war.[21]

Into 2025 – during that moment or year of reflection – the 'Nimbus' (NB.1.8.1) co-circulating variant of Omicron had shown itself to be growing as a proportion of all coronavirus cases internationally, and the 'Stratus' (subvariant XFG) followed on too. In Sweden, cases of coronavirus had risen from 6,000 to 30,000 daily. Magnus Gisslén, the country's state epidemiologist since 2023 – successor to Tegnell and Lindblom – said that it was 'not impossible that there could be an increased spread of infection during the summer and autumn'. The WHO had been 'keeping an extra eye' on the 'Nimbus' mutation that had been first discovered in Asia, where it had been spreading like wildfire. The mutation had become a variant under monitoring (VUM) by public health authorities, one that required prioritized attention.[22]

Sweden had 'long since returned to normality', Forssmed had remarked, and part of that return had been the revoking or abolition during the short Andersson administration of legacy enactments in wake of the coronavirus crisis. The temporary Pandemic Law which had been extended until January 2022, as well as the temporary infection control measures to limit the spread of COVID-19 in bars and restaurants had expired by 31 March 2022. Then, as of 1 April 2022, the *Riksdag* voted to declassify COVID-19 as a reportable contagious disease.[23]

While Sweden had much to do in addressing the shortcomings exposed by the *Coronakommission* – some of which had been addressed by Forssmed – in the wider world too there had been much to be done, not least with regard to an international pandemic treaty, and the ongoing COVAX global vaccine programme.

In March 2021, world leaders had announced an initiative for a new treaty on pandemic preparedness and response. The initiative was taken to the WHO where a draft was negotiated and debated. The world's first Pandemic Agreement would not be reached until May 2025 and the gathering of the 78th World Health Assembly in Geneva.[24]

Delegates at the 77th meeting in 2024 had said that further negotiations would be needed. WHO member states had reached agreement on several areas during that meeting, but there remained serious differences on finance, and how much pharmaceutical product would be set aside for countries in need, as well as on intellectual property rights and sanctions.[25] These differences had clearly been settled.

In March 2023, the Swedish government announce that 722,000 doses of the Pfizer/BioNTech COVID-19 vaccine would be donated to the COVAX global vaccine initiative. In so doing, Sweden had donated more than 15 million doses and contributed more than SEK 2 billion to global vaccination effort against the virus. By then, some 72 per cent of the world's population had received at least one dose of vaccine, though in low-income countries the number was just 23 per cent. In total, 13.2 billion vaccine doses had been administered globally.[26]

By the time that the final report of the *Coronakommission* had been published, academic studies had shown that Sweden was likely to have done much better than other countries in terms of the economy, education, mental health, and domestic abuse, and that it had come through the pandemic with less excess mortality than in almost any other European country. Additionally, it was less than half that of the USA, the very same country where Donald Trump and major media outlets had repeatedly used Sweden as a cautionary tale – 'You did not want to be like Sweden'. It might be argued though that it had not been Sweden engaging in a reckless, unprecedented pandemic experiment, but the rest of the world, and without any evidence of the sense of implementing drastic lockdowns. Maybe Sweden's *laissez-faire* (*låt det vara*) approach had paid off.[27] Imagine that.

So then, Sweden, foolhardy or exceptional, pariah or paragon, the reader had been asked in the Introduction to this book. Perhaps Sweden had been not so much a 'misfit', 'maverick', 'outlier', 'pariah', or 'paragon', but rather a country whose approach or strategy was 'principled', with principles based on its own rules and on its own tried and tested system of governance – Sweden in the role of defiant and independent Pippi Longstocking perhaps. All until a 'real' crisis struck anyway, and the *Coronakommission* spotlighted the need to question that governance.

And finally, after the initial fraught two years of COVID-19 among us, how many people had died, say, to 2025? Across the world, by August 2025, there had been 7,099,056 cumulative confirmed deaths. Across the continents, in Europe,

2,109,261 people had died, in North America 1,704,907, in Asia 1,637,870, in South America 1,355,560, in Africa 258,288, and in Oceania 33,170.[28]

Across the twenty-seven countries of the European Union, 1,268,589 people had died. In the Nordic region, cumulative deaths in Sweden amounted to 28,849 which had been a slight jump since March, in Finland 11,466, in Denmark 10,012, in Norway 5,732, Iceland 186, Faroe Islands 28, and Greenland 21.

In Hungary, which was slightly smaller than Sweden, 49,124 cumulative deaths had been recorded by August 2025. Slightly larger than Sweden population-wise, to various degrees, were Belgium, Greece, Czechia, and Portugal, each suffering more cumulative deaths than Sweden. In Czechia, 43,816 deaths had been recorded; in Greece, 40,086; in Belgium 34,339; and in Portugal, 29,359.[29]

Cumulative deaths in the USA to August 2025 were 1,226,351, in Brazil 703,051, in India 533,837, in Russia 404,290, in the UK 232,112, and in China 122,398. Italy had experienced 198,523 deaths by August 2025, Germany had 174,979, France 168,162, Spain 121,852, Poland 120,978, the Netherlands 22,986, Austria 22,534, Switzerland 14,170, and Ireland 9,848. The Cook Islands and Saint Pierre and Miquelon had two deaths, Nauru and Tuvalu 1, and the Falkland Islands, Niue, Pitcairn, Saint Helena, Tokelau, Turkmenistan, and Vatican City 0. North Korea also claimed to have had none.[30]

Notes

1 Oscarsson, Henrik *et al. Väljarna och valet 2022*, Valforsknings-programmet, No. 186, Göteborg Studies in Politics, p. 38, p. 43, p. 52, p. 54.

2 Löfven was born in Stockholm in 1957 but before he was even one-year old he began a new life growing up in Sunnersta in Ådalen, in Ångermanland, in the north of Sweden, as the foster child of Iris (1929–2020) and Ture Melander (1926–2003). Löfven's foster- father was a factory worker, and earlier a lumberjack, and his foster-mother was a care visitor to the elderly in their district.

3 Löfven, Stefan. i samarbete med Ulrika Knutson. *Svetsare och statsminister*, p. 171

4 'Karin Tegmark Wisell appointed as Sweden's ambassador for global health', Ministry of Health and Social Affairs, Press release, Government Offices of Sweden, 9 July 2024, <http://www.government.se/press-releases/2024/07/karin-tegmark-wisell-apppointed-as-swedens-ambassador-for-global-health/> accessed 22 January 2025.

5 Kleja, Monica. 'Presenterades i mars – nu ska nya statsepidemiologen sluta. Tidigare smittskyddsläkaren Anders Lindblom kommer att sluta sin nya tjänst som statsepidemiolog den 30 juni', *Dagens Medicin*, 6 April 2022, <https://www.dagensmedicin.se/arbetsliv/personnytt/presenterades-i-mars-nu-ska-nya-statsepidemiolog-sluta#> accessed 31 January 2025.

6 Habib, Heba. 'Has Sweden's controversial covid-19 strategy been successful?' *Medical Journal, BMJ*, 12 June 2020, updated 18 June 2020, <https://doi.org/10.1136/bmj.m2376> accessed 31 January 2025.

7 Ahlander, Johan. 'Sweden saw lower 2020 death spike than much of Europe – data', *Reuters*, 24 March 2021, <https://www.reuters.com/article/us-health-coronavirus-europe-mortality-idUSKBN2BG1R9/> accessed 17 January 2025.

8 Ibid.
9 Norberg, Johan. 'Sweden during the pandemic. Pariah or paragon?' p. 7, *CATO policy analysis*, No. 959, 29 August 2023, Cato Institute, <https://www.cato.org/sites/cato.org/files/2023-08/policy-analysis-959-no-link.pdf> accessed 6 February 2025.
10 'Comparisons of all-cause mortality between European countries and regions: 28 December 2019 to week ending 1 July 2022', Office for National Statistics, <https://www.ons.gov.uk/peoplepopulationandcommunity/birthsdeathsandmarriages/ deaths/articles/comparisomofallcausemortalitybetweeneuropeancountriesandregions/ 28december2019toweekending1july2022> accessed 17 January 2025.
11 'Excess mortality: Cumulative deaths from all causes compared to projection based on previous years, per million people, Dec 31, 2020, and Dec 31, 2023', Our World in Data, COVID-19 dataset, <https://ourworldindata.org> accessed 7 February 2025.
12 Ahlander, as note 7.
13 Witness statement of Professor Anders Tegnell. Statement No.1, Exhibit AT/001, UK Covid-19 Inquiry, 2 October 2023, <https://covid19.public-inquiry.uk/wp-content/uploads/2023/12/18145343/INQ000283502.pdf> accessed 16 January 2025.
14 Terms of reference of the UK Covid-19 Inquiry, and detail concerning 'Every story matters', <https://covid19.public-inqiry.uk/documents/terms-of-reference/> and <https://covid19.public-inquiry.uk/every-story-matters/> accessed 15 January 2025. Chair of the UK Covid-19 Inquiry, the Rt. Hon. Baroness Heather Carol Hallet DBE, conducted the inquest of those who died in the 7 July 2005 London bombings.
15 Witness statement of Professor Anders Tegnell, Point 27, Point 48, Point 52, Point 64– 66, Point 68 in the testimony.
16 'Inquiry chair meets Sweden's former state epidemiologist', Scottish Covid-19 Inquiry, <https://covid19inquiry.scot/news/inquiry-chair-meets-swedens-former-state-epidemiologist> accessed 16 January 2025.
17 Baldwin, Peter. 'Sweden stumbles along the third way', in Sigurd Bergman, and Martin Lindström, *Sweden's pandemic experiment*, 2022, p. 2.
18 Ibid.
19 Opinion piece by Minister for Social Affairs and Public Health Jakob Forssmed, Altinget, Politik på allvar, 4 February 2025, <https://www.regeringen.se/debattartiklar/2025/02/forssmed-vi-far-inte-glomma-coronapandemins-lardomar/> accessed 19 May 2025.
20 Ibid.
21 Ibid.
22 'Ny covidvariant sprids – fall i Sverige', Senaste nyheterna i korthet, *Dagens Nyheter*, 9 June 2025, <https://www.dn.se/dirkt/2025-06-09/ny-covidvariant-sprids-fall-i-sverige/> and, 'Larmet: Nimbus har nått Sverige: Kan ha muterat', *Aftonbladet*, 14 June 2025, <https://www.aftonbladet.se/nyheter/a/QM4vwP/ny-covidvariant-sprids-lavinartat-har-natt-sverige> and, 'Should we be worried about the new COVID-19 variant?' Blog, UK Health Security Agency, 13 May 2024, updated June 2025. and, 'WHO TAG-VE risk evaluation for SARS-CoV-2 variant under monitoring: NB.1.8.1', World Health Organization, WHO, 23 May 2025, <https://cdn.who.int/media/docs/default-source/documents/epp/tracking-sars-cov-2/23052025_nb.1.8.1_ire.pdf> accessed 13 June 2025.
23 'Sweden: Parliament revokes COVID-19 emergency legislation', Article, Library of Congress, <https://www.loc.gov/item/global-legal-monitor/2022-03-29/sweden-parliament-revokes-covid-19-emergency-legislation/> accessed 19 May 2025.
24 Butchard, Patrick. and Bukky Balogun. 'What is the WHO Pandemic Treaty?' House of Commons Library, 29 May 2024, <https://researchbriefings.files.parliament.uk/documents/CBP-9550/CBP-9550.pdf> accessed 20 January 2025, and, 'World Health Assembly adopts historic Pandemic Agreement to make the world more equitable and safer from future

pandemics', News release, WHO, 20 May 2025, <https://www.who.int/news/item/20-05-2025-world-health-assembly-adopts-historic-pandemic-agreement-to-make-the-world-more-equitable-and-safer-from-future-pandemics> accessed 22 May 2025.

25 Lay, Kat. 'Global pandemic treaty could be more than a year away after deadline missed', *The Guardian*, 29 May 2024, <https://www.theguardian.com/global-development/article/2024/may/29/global- pandemic-treaty-could-be-more-than-a-year-away-after-deadline-missed> accessed 20 January 2025.

26 'The Swedish government is donating 722 million COVID-19 vaccine doses to low- and middle-income countries', Ministry for Foreign Affairs, Press release, Government Offices of Sweden, 1 March 2023, <https://www.government.se/press-releases/2023/03/government-donating-722-000-million-covid-19-vaccine-doses-to-low--and-middle-income-countries/> accessed 23 January 2025.

27 Norberg, as note 9, p. 10, p. 11.

28 'Cumulative confirmed COVID-19 deaths ', Our World in Data Dataset, updated data extracted to 10 August 2025, <https://ourworldindata.org/grapher/cumulative-deaths-and-cases-covid-19?tab=table&time=2021-02-26..latest> accessed 2 September 2025.

29 Ibid.

30 Ibid.

Bibliography

Abzhandadze, Tamar *et al.*, 'Sick leave one year after Covid-19 infection: a nationwide cohort study during the first wave in Sweden', *Scientific reports*, 14, 572 (January 2024).

Ahlander, Johan. 'Sweden saw lower 2020 death spike than much of Europe – data', *Reuters* (24 March 2021).

Ahlander, Johan, and Simon Johnson, 'Sweden should have done more against coronavirus but broad strategy right: chief epidemiologist', *Reuters* (3 June 2020).

Baldwin, Peter, 'Sweden stumbles along the third way', in Sigurd Bergman, and Martin Lindström, *Sweden's pandemic experiment*, (Routledge 2022).

Ball, Philip, 'Ten lessons of the pandemic', *New Statesman*, pp.23–27 (23–29 October 2020).

Baynes, Chris, 'Coronavirus pandemic will be lengthy, World Health Organisation warns', *The Independent* (2 August 2020).

Bendjelloul, Johar, and Jonas Lindkvist, 'Folkhälsomyndighetens Johan Carlson: Det är klart att det kan kännas lite skrämmande', *Dagens Nyheter* (5 April 2020).

Bergan, Ronald, 'Petter Lindstrom', *The Guardian* (17 June 2000).

Birnbaum, Norman, 'Portrait of a Swedish town', *New York Times* (24 September 1972).

Biswas, Soutik. 'What is the Indian COVID variant and will vaccines work?' *BBC News (23 April 2021).*

Bjarnefors, Stefan, and Amanda Dahl, 'WHO: Smittspridningen stabil i Sverige', *Dagens Nyheter* (26 June 2020)

Bjurwald, Lisa, 'Opinion: I believe Sweden will regret its approach to COVID in schools', *The Local* (16 August 2021).

Bratt, Anna, 'Därför stoppas bara Modernas vaccin', *Dagens Nyheter* (6 October 2021, updated 7 October 2021).

Brown, Joe David, 'Swedish sin', *Time* (Atlantic edition), 65, no.17 (25 April 1955).

Butchard, Patrick. and Bukky Balogun, 'What is the WHO Pandemic Treaty?' House of Commons Library, Research Briefing (29 May 2024).

Carp, Ossi, 'Norge ger klartecken för ytterligare fyra Svenska regioner', *Dagens Nyheter (24 July 2020).*

Carp, Ossi, and Amanda Lindholm, and Alexandra Carlsson Tenitskaja. 'En gripen och etttiotal brottsmisstänkta efter anti-coronademonstration i Stockholm', *Dagens Nyheter (1 May 2021).*

Christensen, Christian, 'Opinion: Why can't foreign media see past Sweden's far-right', *The Local (2 July 2021)*

Christiansson, Magnus, 'Chapter II. The NATO question in Sweden under the Trump presidency – Military non-alignment between power politics and feminist foreign policy', in *Finland, Sweden & NATO. Did Trump change everything*, Jaan Siitonen, pp. 39–55 (Helsinki: Svenska bildningsförbundet SBF, 2017).

Crace, John, 'Out in the cold', an interview with Roland Huntford, *The Guardian* (27 December 2008).

Cursino, Malu, 'COVID: Germany tightens restrictions on UK travellers', *BBC News* (20 December 2021).

Cuthbertson, Anthony, 'Coronavirus tracked: Charting Sweden's disastrous no-lockdown strategy', *Independent* (1 June 2020).

Dahl, Amanda, 'Skarp kritik mot svensk coronahantering: Otillräckliga åtgärder', *Dagens Nyheter (29 October 2021).*

Delin, Michael, and Hanna Jakobson, 'Dan Eliasson i KU: MSB ville larma tidigare', *Dagens Nyheter* (26 March 2021).

Duxbury, Charlie, 'How Sweden's prime minister plans to save his career from coronavirus' Politico.eu (24 December 2020).

Eaton, George, 'Trust is vital if you want to stop this disease', Anders Tegnell on leading Sweden's fight against Covid-19, *New Statesman*, (23–29 October 2020).

Edwards, Catherine, 'As Europe comes out of lockdown, what lessons can be learned from Sweden?' *The Local* (20 May 2020).

Edwards, Catherine, 'Sweden's Anders Tegnell questioned over strategy and errors', *The Local*, 3 June 2020,

Edwards, Catherine, 'Is it right to say Sweden is still not experiencing a second wave of COVID-19', *The Local* (16 October 2020).

Edwards, Catherine, 'Analysis: Is Sweden heading for a national lockdown?', *The Local (6 November 2020).*

Edwards, Catherine, 'Explained: The five new coronavirus measures that Sweden just announced', *The Local* (17 February 2021).

Edwards, Catherine, 'How concerned should we be about the spread of the Delta COVID-19 variant in Sweden?', *The Local* (17 June 2021).

Ekeblad, Matilda, Förbundsordförande MUF, 'Misslyckandet är totalt – avgå, Lena Hallengren', *Expressen* (20 December 2020).

Emanuelsson, Eric, and Max Sohl Stjernberg, 'Gun-Britt Johnsson, 91, först i Sverige med attfå vaccin', *Expressen* (27 December 2020).

Eriksson, Aleksandra, 'Sweden fights back as foreign leaders make up bad news', Eurobserver.com (20 February 2017).

European Centre for Disease Prevention and Control, 'Overview of COVID-19 vaccination strategies and vaccine deployment in the EU/EEA and the UK', Technical report, 2 December 2020 (Stockholm/Solna: ECDC, 2020).

European Commission, 'Europe's moment: Repair and prepare for the next generation', Press release, 27 May 2020 (Brussels: European Commission, 2020).

European Commission, 'Questions & answers on the coordination of measures restricting free movement in the European Union related to the coronavirus pandemic', Press corner, 13 October 2020 (Brussels: European Commission, 2020).

European Commission, 'EU Digital COVID Certificate: European Parliament and Council reach agreement on Commission proposal', Press release, 20 May 2021 (Brussels: European Commission, 2021).

European Council / Council of the European Union, 'Employment, Social Policy, Health and Consumer Affairs Council (Health'), Meetings, 13 February 2020 (Brussels: European Council / Council of the European Union, 2020).

European Council / Council of the European Union, 'COVID-19 outbreak: the presidency steps up EU response by triggering full activation mode of IPCR', Press release, 2 March 2020 (Brussels: European Council / Council of the European Union, 2020).

European Council / Council of the European Union, 'A roadmap for recovery. Towards a more resilient, sustainable and fair Europe', 21 April 2020 (Brussels: European Council / Council of the European Union, 2020).

European Council / Council of the European Union, 'Conclusions of the President of the European Council following the video conference of the members of the European Council, 23 April 2020', 23 April 2020 (Brussels: European Council / Council of the European Union, 2020).

European Council / Council of the European Union, 'Council agrees to start lifting travel restrictions for residents of some third countries', Press release, 30 June 2020 (Brussels: European Council / Council of the European Union, 2020).

European Council / Council of the European Union, 'An international treaty on pandemicprevention and preparedness', 30 March 2021 (Brussels: European Council / Council of the European Union, 2021).

Ewald, Hugo, and Hans Olsson, 'Stefan Löven i karantän', *Dagens Nyheter* (6 November 2020).

Farmbrough, Heather, 'Why Sweden's approach to coronavirus may not be what you think', *Forbes* (14 May 2020).

Florida, Richard. and Charlotta Mellander, 'The geography of COVID-19 in Sweden', *The annals of regional science, Vol. 68, pp. 125–150 (2022).*

Folkhälsomyndigheten / Public Health Agency, 'Veckorapport on covid-19, vecka 15 (a report taken over 6–12 April 2020, week 15)', 17 April 2020 (Stockholm/ Solna: Folkhälsomyndigheten, 2020).

Folkhälsomyndigheten / Public Health Agency, 'FAQ about COVID-19', 8 December 2020 (Stockholm/Solna: Folkhälsomyndigheten, 2020).

Forrest, Adam, 'Boris Johnson pursuing COVID policy of mass infection that poses danger to the world, scientists warn', *The Independent* (16 July 2021).

Forrest, Adam, 'WHO calls for ban on sale of live animals in food markets to combat pandemics', *The Independent* (13 April 2021).

Foster, Alice, 'Sweden and Donald Trump: the controversy explained', *Express* (20 February 2017).

Foster, Keith, 'US President Trump says Sweden is suffering in the corona crisis', Sveriges Radio (11 April 2020).

Franke, Peter, 'Se dig själv i spegeln, Ebba',*VF, Värmlands Folkblad* (8 June 2020).

Franssen, Anne Grietje, 'Why are there so many coronavirus cases in Stockholm's northern suburbs?' *The Local* (9 April 2020).

Gallagher, James, 'New COVID variant: How worried should we be?' *BBC News* (26 November 2021).

Garcia, Carmen Aguilar, and Ganesh Rao, 'COVID-19: India's vaccine export ban could send shockwaves worldwide. Should the UK step in to help?', Sky News (30 April 2021).

Gonzalez, Ana Espinosa, and Elina Suzuki, 'The impacts of long Covid across OECD countries' OECD Health Working Papers, No. 167 (13 June 2024).

Gorokov, S. A. *et al.*, 'Little Mogadishu in Stockholm, or Apartheid with a friendly face in Sweden', pp. 57–65, Asia & Africa today, No. 3 (Moscow: Russian Centre for Scientific Information, 2024).

Haager, Julia Sophie. 'What makes Pippi Longstocking a classic of identity empowerment?' Televizion, 29/2016/E, 22 May 2016 (Munich: IZI, 2016).

Habib, Heba, 'Has Sweden's controversial covid-19 strategy been successful?' *British Medical Journal, BMJ (12 June 2020, updated 18 June 2020).*

Habib, Heba, 'COVID-19: What Sweden taught Scandinavia for the second wave', *British Medical Journal, BMJ (27 November 2020).*

Hale, Frederick, 'Challenging the Swedish social welfare state: the case of Dwight D. Eisenhower', in Swedish-American Historical Quarterly, v. 54, no. 1, pp.55-71 (January 2003).

Hancock, Sam, 'AstraZeneca vaccine: No evidence to restrict use of Covid jab, says EMA boss says', The Independent (31 March 2021).

Hansson, Erik *et al.*, 'Million-dollar program, migrants, and vulnerability to COVID-19', Delmi Policy Brief 2021:2 (Stockholm: Delegationen för Migrationsstudier, 2021).

Henley, Jon, 'Global report: France could lose control of Covid-19 at any time', *The Guardian (4 August 2020).*

Henley, Jon, 'Decomposing mink in Denmark may have contaminated groundwater', *The Guardian* (10 December 2020).
Henley, Jon, 'EU may not renew vaccine contract with AstraZeneca over delivery shortfalls', *The Guardian* (19 April 2021).
Herold, Lovis, 'Kraftig ökning av antalet covid-19-fall i Västra Götalandsregionen', *Dagens Nyheter* (4 June 2020).
Holm, Gusten, 'Professorn: Sverige kan få Italiens situation', *Expressen* (15 March 2020).
Holm, Gusten, and Max Stohl Stjernberg, and Daniel Ingmo, 'Bilderna avslöjar: Här julbesöker Löfven Gallerian', *Expressen* (9 December 2020).
Holmgren Mia, 'Tegnell: Största utmaningen är att nå ut med relevant information om Astras vaccin', *Dagens Nyheter* (20 April 2021).
Irwin, Rachel Elisabeth, 'Misinformation and de-contextualization: international media reporting on Sweden and COVID-19', *Globalization and health*, 16, 2020 (13 July 2020).
Jakobson, Hanna, and Amanda Dahl, 'KU: Regeringen har brustit i hanteringen av pandemin', *Dagens Nyheter* (3 June 2021).
James, Liam, 'What is mink-related coronavirus?' *Independent* (7 November 2020).
Karlsten, Emanuel, 'Mejlen som avslöjar Gieseckes inflytande', *Expressen* (11 August 2020).
Kleja, Monica, 'Presenterades i mars – nu ska nya statsepidemiologen sluta. Tidigare smittskyddsläkaren Anders Lindblom kommer att sluta sin nya tjänst som statsepidemiolog den 30 juni', *Dagens Medicin* (6 April 2022).
Kungl. Vetenskapsakademien / Royal Swedish Academy of Sciences, 'Ny rapport om munskydd och ventilation från Vetenskapsakademiens expertgrupp om Covid-19', Press release, 19 November 2020 (Stockholm: Kungl. Vetenskapsakademien, 2020).
Lagerwall, Katerina, and Amanda Dahl, 'WHO backar delvis om Sverige som högriskland', Dagens Nyheter (26 June 2020).
Lagerwall, Katarina, 'Fler minkbesättningar i Sverige smittade av coronavirus', *Dagens Nyheter (5 November 2020).*
Lallerstedt, Siri, 'Det här är pandemilagen och tillfälliga serveringslag', *Dagens Nyheter* (12 August 2021).
Lawton, Graham, 'Is a dangerous new coronavirus strain circulating in farmed mink?' *New Scientist* (6 November 2020).
Lay, Kat, 'Global pandemic treaty could be more than a year away after deadline missed', *The Guardian* (29 May 2024).
Lichfield, John, 'Opinion: European governments were cautious on AstraZeneca vaccines but they were neither stupid nor political', *The Local* (19 March 2021).
Linder, Julia, and Sofia Tanaka, and Mia Holmgren, 'FHM:s nya riktlinjer efter första november: Vaccinerade behöver inte testa sig', *Dagens Nyheter* (14 October 2021).

Löfgren, Emma, 'The biggest challenge of our time: How Sweden doubled intensive care capacity amid COVID-19 panic', *The Local* (23 June 2020).

Löfgren, Emma, 'Sweden announces new exceptions to non-EU travel ban', *The Local (2 July 2020).*

Löfgren, Emma, 'New coronavirus measures rolled out in three Swedish regions, including Stockholm and Gothenburg', *The Local* (29 October 2020).

Löfgren, Emma, 'Sweden rolls out series of new coronavirus measures, including face masks', *The Local* (18 December 2020).

Löfgren, Emma, 'Sweden in violation of EU law for failing to issue COVID passes to thousands of foreign residents', *The Local* (25 August 2021, updated 29 August 2021).

Löfven, Stefan, i samarbete med Ulrika Knutson. *Svetsare och statsminister* (Stockholm: Atlas 2024).

Looi, Mun-Keat, 'Covid-19: Is a second wave hitting Europe?' *British Medical Journal*, BMJ (28 October 2020).

Lundberg, Patrik, 'Nu firar vi medelklassens frihetsdag', *Dagens Nyheter* (28 September 2021).

Mackenzie, Jean, 'How Iceland clamped down to conquer coronavirus', *BBC News* (23 March 2021)

Mallapaty, Smriti, 'COVID mink analysis shows mutations are not dangerous – yet', *Nature*, No. 587, pp. 340–41 (13 November 2020).

Marr, Andrew, interviewing Isabella Lövin, *Andrew Marr Show*, BBC (Sunday 26 April 2020).

Merklund, Carl, 'From false neutrality to true socialism: US Sweden-bashing during the later Palme years, 1973-1986', in *The journal of transnational American studies*, vol.7, issue 1 (2016).

Merklund, Carl, 'Därför beskrivs Sverige som en dystopi', *Dagens Nyheter* (21 February 2017).

Milford, Chiara, 'Five of Sweden's regions open COVID-19 vaccine booking to all over-18s', *The Local* (30 June 2021).

Milne, Robert, 'Sweden: why the moral superpower dissented over COVID-19', *Financial Times (16 October 2020).*

Murphy, Flynn, 'Inside China's response to COVID', *Nature*, No. 588, pp. 49–51 (2 December 2020).

Muri, Karin, and Janne Møller-Hansen, 'Må bare si fra', *VG*, *Verdens Gang* (20 December 2020).

Nelson, Fraser, 'Sweden tames its R number without lockdown', *The Spectator* (4 May 2020).

NIH, 'New coronavirus emerges from bats in China, devastates young swine', 4 April 2018 (Bethesda MD: National Institutes of Health, 2018).

Norberg, Johan, 'Sweden during the pandemic. Pariah or paragon?' *CATO policy analysis*, No. 959, 29 August 2023 (Washington, D.C.: Cato Institute, 2023).

Norwell, Frazer, 'Oslo to Gothenburg train service set to make a return', *The Local* (3 September 2021).

Nygren, Katarina Giritli, and Anna Olofsson, 'Swedish exceptionalism, herd immunity and the welfare state: A media analysis of struggles over the nature and legitimacy of the Covid-19 pandemic strategy in Sweden', *Sociology, gender studies and cultural studies*, Vol. 69. No. 4, pp. 529–546 (2021).

OECD, 'Tackling coronavirus (COVID-19). Contributing to a global effort. Sweden. Containment measures', 15 April 2020 (Paris: OECD, 2020).

O'Leary, Naomi, 'Sweden and coronavirus: how has the outlier of Europe fared?' *The Irish Times (23 September 2020).*

Olsson, Gustav, 'Gävleborg pausar Moderna helt—behöver inte längre vaccinet', *Dagens Nyheter (7 October 2021).*

Olsson, Gustav. 'Världen passerar fem miljoner dödsfall – rika länder hårt drabbade', *Dagens Nyheter* (1 November 2021).

Olsson, Gustav, and Amanda Dahl, 'Sverige går emot ökande smittotrend i Europa', Dagens Nyheter (28 July 2020).

Orange, Richard, 'Why is everyone in Sweden talking about Anders Tegnell's emails?' *The Local (12 August 2020).*

Orange, Richard, 'Muppets and free love: The bizarre documentary that shaped the image of Sweden', *The Local* (12 March 2021).

Oscarsson, Henrik *et al.*, *Väljarna och valet 2022*, Valforsknings-programmet, No. 186, *Göteborg Studies in Politics* (Göteborgs universitet, 2024).

Pancevski, Bojan, 'German infectiologist Ansgar Lohse joins experts who say [...]' [Twitter post] @bopanc, 29 March 2020, accessed 4 June 2020.

Pancevski, Bojan, and Dominic Chopping, 'Inside Sweden's radically different approach to the coronavirus', *The Wall Street Journal* (30 March 2020).

Parkes, Brandon *et al.*, 'Community factors and excess mortality in the COVID-19 pandemic in England, Italy and Sweden', *European journal of public health*, Vol. 33, No. 4, pp. 695–703 (2023).

Picheta, Rob, 'The UK has more Covid-19 cases than France, Germany, Italy and Spain combined', CNN (21 October 2021).

Poole, Steven, 'Word of the week: who benefits from herd immunity', *The Guardian* (14 October 2020).

Rapacioli, Paul, *Good Sweden, bad Sweden: The use and abuse of Swedish values in a post-truth world (Stockholm: Volante, 2018).*

Rapacioli, Paul, 'When a US president speaks about Sweden, the fallout can last a long time', *The Local* (12 January 2018).

Ray, John, 'Is Sweden's decision not to have a coronavirus lockdown a fatal mistake?' ITV News (29 April 2020).

Reicher, Stephen, 'Johnson has ignored the science and blown our chance to stop a second wave', *The Guardian* (13 October 2020).

Rosén, Hans, 'Alla med symptom ska testas – regeringen satsar 6 miljarder', *Dagens Nyheter (4 June 2020).*

Rothschild, Natalie, 'The hidden flaws in Sweden's anti-lockdown strategy', *Foreign Policy (21 April 2020).*
Savage, Maddy, 'Could the Swedish lifestyle help fight coronavirus?' BBC, Remote Control. Covid-19 (28 March 2020).
Schlessinger, June H., 'Pippi Longstocking by Astrid Lindgren', Research Starters Home (EBSCO, 2022).
Shearing, Hazel, 'COVID: UK faces a difficult summer, says leading scientist', *BBC News* (18 July 2021).
Shin, Qing *et al.*, 'Covid-19 illness severity and 2-year prevalence of physical symptoms: an observational study in Iceland, Sweden, Norway and Denmark', The Lancet Regional Health – Europe, Volume 35, 100756 (October 2023).
Simons, Gregg, 'Swedish government and country image during the international media coverage of the coronavirus pandemic strategy: from bold to pariah', in *Journalism and media*, 1 (1), pp. 41–58, 12 November 2020 (Basel: Multidisciplinary Digital Publishing Institute, MDPI, 2020).
Siitonen, Jaan, *Finland, Sweden & NATO. Did Trump change everything* (Helsinki: Svenska bildningsförbundet SBF, 2017).
Sokolnicki, Amanda, 'Moderaternas roll i pandemin är ingenting att vara stolt över', *Dagens Nyheter (19 December 2020).*
Stenberg, Ewa, 'Löfven pressas allt mer i coronakrisen', *Dagens Nyheter* (4 June 2020).
Stenberg, Ewa, 'Därför har väljarna inte get Löfven skulden', *Dagens Nyheter* (27 April 2021).
Stenberg, Ewa, 'Hallengren har en del att ångra – trots allt', *Dagens Nyheter* (30 October 2021).
Stenberg, Ewa, 'Svårt att utkräva politiskt ansvar för dödsfallen', *Dagens Nyheter* (25 February 2022).
Svahn, Clas, 'Sverige kan ha modifierat vaccin inom tre månader', *Dagens Nyheter* (26 November 2021, updated 27 November 2021).
Swedish Government Official Reports, 'Äldreomsorgen under pandemin'. Delbetänkande av Coronakommissionen, English Summary, Statens Offentliga Utredningar SOU 2020:80, Stockholm, 7 December 2020 (Stockholm: Government Offices of Sweden, 2020).
Swedish Government Official Reports, 'Sverige under pandemin'. Volym 1 'Smittspridning och smittskydd'. Volym 2 'Sjukvård och folkhälsa'. Delbetänkande 2 / Interim Repor 2. Coronakommissionen, Summary in English. Statens Offentliga Utredningar SOU 2021:89, Stockholm, 29 October 2021 (Stockholm: Government Offices of Sweden, 2021).
Swedish Government Official Reports,'Sverige under pandemin'. Volym 1 'Samhällets, företagens och enskildas ekonomi'. Volym 2 'Förutsättningar, vägval ochutvärdering'. Slutbetänkande av Coronakommissionen. Summary in English. Statens Offentliga Utredningar SOU 2022:10, Stockholm, 25 February 2022 (Stockholm: Government Offices of Sweden, 2022).

Swedish Government Press Information, 'How Sweden is governed. Public agencies and how they are governed. Ministerial rule prohibited in Sweden', 2 March 2015 (Stockholm: Government Offices of Sweden, 2015).

Swedish Ministry for Foreign Affairs, 'Statement of Government Policy by Minister for Foreign Affairs, Ann Linde, in the Parliamentary Debate on foreign affairs, Wednesday 24 February 2021 (Stockholm: Government Offices of Sweden, 2021).

Swedish Ministry of Foreign Affairs, 'The Swedish government is donating 722 million COVID-19 vaccine doses to low- and middle-income countries', Press release, 1 March2023 (Stockholm: Government Offices of Sweden, 2023)

Swedish Ministry of Health and Social Affairs, 'Mats Melin to chair COVID-19 inquiry in Sweden', 1 July 2020 (Stockholm: Government Offices of Sweden, 2020).

Swedish Ministry of Health and Social Affairs, 'E-hälsomyndigheten ska undersöka om flervaccinerade grupper kan fä covidbevis', 26 August 2021 (Stockholm: Government Offices of Sweden, 2021).

Swedish Ministry of Health and Social Affairs, 'Utredning ska se över smittskyddslagen införframtida pandemier', Press release, 31 August 2021 (Stockholm: Government Offices of Sweden, 2021).

Swedish Ministry of Health and Social Affairs, 'Några smittskyddsfrågor inom socialtjänstenoch socialförsäkringen, SOU 2023:56, Press release from the Ministry of Health, 19 September 2023, (Stockholm: Government Offices of Sweden, 2023).

Swedish Ministry of Health and Social Affairs, 'Karin Tegmark Wisell appointed as Sweden's ambassador for global health', Press release, 9 July 2024 (Stockholm: Government Offices of Sweden, 2024).

Swedish Ministry of Health and Social Affairs, Opinion piece by Minister for Social Affairs and Public Health Jakob Forssmed, *Altinget, Politik på allvar*, 4 February 2025 (Stockholm: Government Offices of Sweden, 2025).

Swedish Ministry of Justice, 'Vaccinated travellers to Sweden from the UK to be exempted from entry ban and test requirement', 7 October 2021 (Stockholm: Government Offices of Sweden, 2021).

Swedish Prime Minister's Office, Statement of Government Policy given by Prime Minister Stefan Löfven before the Riksdag, 8 September 2020 (Stockholm: Government Offices of Sweden, 2020).

Swedish Prime Minister's Office, 'Prime Minister Stefan Löfven's address to the nation', 22 November 2020 (Stockholm: Government Offices of Sweden, 2020).

Tanaka, Sofia, and Gustav Olsson, 'Lägre andel bland utlandsfödda som vaccinerar sig', *Dagens Nyheter* (29 April 2021).

Treijs, Erica, and Eric Olsson, 'Suhonen: Kanske måste Löfven offra Hallengren', *Svenska Dagbladet (20 December 2020).*

Triggle, Nick, 'Covid: The UK is Europe's virus hotspot – does it matter?', *BBC News* (9 October 2021).

UK Covid-19 Inquiry, 'Witness statement of Professor Anders Tegnell'. Statement No.1,Exhibit AT/001, UK COVID-19 Inquiry (2 October 2023).

UN Office for the Coordination of Humanitarian Affairs (OCHA), 'UN welcomes nearly $1 billion in recent pledges – to bolster access to lifesaving tests, treatments and vaccines to end COVID-19', reliefweb, 30 September 2020 (New York: UN/OCHA, 2020).

US Congress, House of Representatives, Committee on Oversight and Accountability, Summary of the 'Final report: COVID select concludes 2-year investigation, issues 500+ page final report on lessons learned and the path forward', Press release, 2 December 2024 (Washington, DC: House Oversight and Accountability Select Subcommittee on the Coronavirus Pandemic, 2024).

Vogel, Gretchen, 'It's been so, so surreal. Critics of Sweden's lax pandemic policies face fierce backlash', *Science*, AAAS.org, 6 October 2020, (American Association for the Advancement of Science, 2020).

Wahlgren, Carl *et al.*, 'Two-year follow-up of patients with post-Covid-19 Condition in Sweden: a prospective cohort study', *The Lancet Regional Health – Europe*, Volume 28, 100595 (May 2023).

Waterton, Becky, 'Swedish politicians call for Covid vaccine pass requirement', *The Local*, (16 November 2021).

Waterton, Becky, 'Which events will require Sweden's new vaccine pass?', *The Local(18 November 2021).*

WHO, 'Statement on the fourth meeting of the International Health Regulations (2005) Emergency Committee regarding the outbreak of coronavirus disease (COVID-19)', 1 August 2020, (Geneva: World Health Organization, 2020).

WHO, 'WHO-convened Global Study of Origins of SARS-CoV-2: China Part', Joint WHO- China Study 14 January-10 February 2021, Joint Report (Geneva: World Health Organization, 2021).

WHO, 'WHO-convened Global Study of Origins of SARS-CoV-2: China Part', Joint WHO- China Study 14 January-10 February 2021, Joint Report, Annex B (Geneva: World Health Organization, 2021).

WHO, 'COVID-19 shows why united action is needed for more robust international health architecture', Commentary, 30 March 2021 (Geneva: World Health Organization, 2021).

WHO, Carl Bildt, former prime Minister of Sweden, appointed WHO Special Envoy for the ACT-Accelerator', News release, 31 March 2021 (Geneva: World Health Organization, 2021).

WHO, 'Classification of Omicron (B.1.1.529): SARS-CoV-2 Variant of Concern', News, 26 November 2021 (Geneva: World Health Organization, 2021).

WHO, 'Statement – Update on COVID-19: Omicron is gaining ground: Protect, prevent, prepare', Statement by Dr. Hans Henri P. Kluge, WHO Regional Director for Europe, Regional Office for Europe, 21 December 2021 (Geneva: World Health Organization, 2021).

WHO, 'World Health Assembly adopts historic Pandemic Agreement to make the world more equitable and safer from future pandemics', News release, 20 May 2025 (Geneva: World Health Organization, 2025).

WHO, 'WHO TAG-VE risk evaluation for SARS-CoV-2 variant under monitoring: NB.1.8.1', 23 May 2025 (Geneva: World Health Organization, 2025).

Winter, Amy Elise, 'The impact of the World Military Games on the COVID-19 pandemic', *Irish journal of medical science*, 190 (4), pp. 1653–1654, 19 January 2021 (Springer / Royal Academy of Medicine in Ireland, 2021).

Woodcock, Andrew, 'Coronavirus: Second wave could last until April in worst case scenario, leaked document reveals', *Independent* (29 October 2020).

Woolhouse, Mark, 'We should follow the Swedes and learn to live with the virus', *The Telegraph* (Sunday 20 September 2020).

Yorke, Harry, and Lucy Fisher, Sarah Knapton, and James Crisp, 'Fury at Emmanuel Macron's nonsense claims about Oxford COVID vaccine', *The Telegraph* (29 January 2021).

Index

The Swedish-language alphabet of 29 letters is composed of the same 26 letters of the English-language plus the vowel modifications Å, Ä, Ö, which appear in that order after the letter Z. However, index terms here which begin with these three letters are simply treated as A, and O.

www.ingramcontent.com/pod-product-compliance
Ingram Content Group UK Ltd.
Pitfield, Milton Keynes, MK11 3LW, UK
UKHW021027041026
15470UKWH00013B/122

9 783034 360777